Interpersonal Communication in Nursing

For Churchill Livingstone:

Commissioning Editor: Susan Young
Project Development Manager: Mairi McCubbin
Project Manager: Joannah Duncan, Pat Miller
Designer: Judith Wright

Interpersonal Communication in Nursing

Theory and Practice

SECOND EDITION

Roger B. Ellis BSc CertEd MEd DipStudCouns
Independent counsellor, psychotherapist and trainer, Lincoln, UK

Bob Gates BEd(Hons) MSc CertEd DipNurs(Lond) RNLD RMN RNT
Head of Learning Disability, Faculty of Health and Human Sciences, Thames Valley University, Berkshire, UK

Neil Kenworthy BEd MBA
Management and training consultant, Lincoln, UK

Illustrations by **Robert Britton** and **Evi Antoniou**

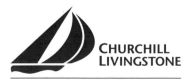

CHURCHILL
LIVINGSTONE

EDINBURGH LONDON NEW YORK OXFORD PHILADELPHIA ST LOUIS SYDNEY TORONTO 2003

CHURCHILL LIVINGSTONE
An imprint of Elsevier Science Limited

©Pearson Professional Limited 1995
©Harcourt Brace and Company Limited 1999
©Harcourt Publishers Limited 2001
©2003, Elsevier Science Limited. All rights reserved.

First published 1995
Second edition 2003

ISBN 0 443 072701

British Library Cataloguing in Publication Data
A catalogue record for this book is available from the British Library

Library of Congress Cataloging in Publication Data
A catalog record for this book is available from the Library of Congress

Notice
Medical knowledge is constantly changing. Standard safety precautions must be followed, but as new research and clinical experience broaden our knowledge, changes in treatment and drug therapy may become necessary or appropriate. Readers are advised to check the most current product information provided by the manufacturer of each drug to be administered to verify the recommended dose, the method and duration of administration, and contraindications. It is the responsibility of the practitioner, relying on experience and knowledge of the patient, to determine dosages and the best treatment for each individual patient. Neither the publisher nor the editors and contributors assume any liability for any injury and/or damage to persons or property arising from this publication.

 ELSEVIER SCIENCE your source for books, journals and multimedia in the health sciences
www.elsevierhealth.com

The publisher's policy is to use **paper manufactured from sustainable forests**

Printed in China

Contents

Contributors

Andy M. Betts MEd RMN AdvDipCouns CertEd CPNCert
Health lecturer, School of Nursing, Lincoln
County Hospital, Lincoln, UK

5 *Improving communication*
7 *The counselling relationship*
9 *Making the most of clinical supervision*

Patricia East BEd (Hons) CertEd MA DipStudCouns
AdvCertPsychotherapy
Independent counsellor and psychotherapist,
Lincoln, UK

8 *The mentoring relationship*
Sadly, Patricia East died in 2000. Her chapter for
this edition has been modified by Roger Ellis.

Roger B. Ellis BSc CertEd MEd DipStudCouns
Independent counsellor and psychotherapist,
Lincoln, UK

1 *Defining communication*
2 *The person in communication*
8 *The mentoring relationship*

Bob Gates BEd(Hons) MSc CertEd DipNurs(Lond) RNLD
RMN RNT
Head of Learning Disability, Faculty of Health
and Human Sciences, Thames Valley University,
Berkshire, UK

2 *The person in communication*

Stuart A. Hindle BSc(Hons) MSc CertEd RGN RMN
RNT RN(USA)
Senior Lecturer, Northumbria University,
Newcastle-upon-Tyne, UK

4 *Psychological factors affecting communication*

Lynda R. Miller MA SRN RMN RNT UKCP
Psychotherapist in private practice, Stromness,
Orkney, UK

6 *Communication in groups and organisations*

Debra Moore BSc(Hons) ENB997 RNMH
Nurse Consultant – Learning Disability, Rampton
Hospital, Trent, UK

11 *Communicating with the wider world*

Peter Morrall BA(Hons) MSc PhD PGCE RN
Senior Lecturer in Health and Sociology,
School of Health, University of Leeds,
Leeds, UK

3 *Social factors affecting communication*

John Turnbull BA MSc RNMH
Director of Nursing and Performance,
Oxfordshire Learning Disability NHS Trust,
Headington, Oxford, UK

10 *Communication and leadership*

Preface

The second edition of this book extends its scope to appeal to nurses at all levels, from diploma and degree students to qualified nurses in clinical and managerial posts. It is also relevant to a wider range of health and social care professions and workers. Ongoing changes in nursing education, together with the ever-widening expectations of health care professionals and the trend for questioning practice, makes it even more imperative that effective communication is developed and maintained between staff, patients and clients, the public and the wider world.

In this second edition the sound basic grounding in fundamental concepts, principles and ideas, and the different theoretical perspectives of communication are retained, as are the practical applications within a range of health care settings which are used to support the theory. It is not just a matter of knowing *about* communication, but also about how we ourselves actually communicate. The contents of this book are therefore intended to enable the reader to make sense of interpersonal communication by reflecting upon it and thereby becoming more objective and analytical. We often take our own ways of communicating for granted so that they go unnoticed by us. By being challenged to examine the ways in which we handle encounters with others, we may develop awareness and insights into our own style of communication and so become more intentional and effective.

The chapters of this book are arranged into two parts. Part 1, 'Foundations of Communication', explores communication and the person; what it is, and why and how individuals communicate. It also looks at factors that influence communication and how communication might be improved. Part 2,

'Communication in Context', contains chapters addressing communication in a number of differing contexts – counselling, leadership, mentoring and clinical supervision, and communication with groups, organisations and the wider world. The chapters on leadership, clinical supervision and communicating with the wider world are new to this second edition, whereas communicating with groups and organisations is an expansion of the first edition.

The editors believe the strengths of this new edition are as follows:

- ◆ It provides a breadth of information for students at pre- and post-professional levels
- ◆ It offers a broad range of communication models
- ◆ It provides the reader with practical examples and assignments in a range of contexts
- ◆ It focuses on the real world of health and social care students and professionals and their communication needs
- ◆ Whilst specifically addressing communication in the field of nursing, the principles and practices are universal – applicable to people whatever their workplace

When nurses achieve insights into the complexities of communication they understand its importance for interpersonal relationships in general and its value in enhancing the quality and success of patient and client care.

Lincoln, 2003

Roger B. Ellis
Bob Gates
Neil Kenworthy

Acknowledgement

The editors wish to give special thanks to Andy Betts who has given generous personal and professional support from the early days of the preparation of this book.

1

Part 1
Foundations of Communication

1

Defining communication

Roger Ellis

DEFINING COMMUNICATION

Human beings have a built-in drive to relate to each other. A baby's very survival depends on getting its caretaker to attend to its needs. The effectiveness and happiness of adults is directly linked to a capacity to form satisfying relationships. The stability and health of any organisation depend on dealing successfully with the complexity of its internal relationships and having effective ways of relating to the outside world. The same applies to nations and countries on the international political scene.

When relationships break down or become a source of stress the central complaint is commonly that of poor communication. 'I just can't get through to my boss. She doesn't seem to want to know what I'm saying'. Often problems in relating stem from the process of communication itself rather than what is being communicated. 'It's not so much what he said but the way he said it that irritated me so much'.

Appeal to common experience bears out these generalisations. Most people have felt anger and helplessness at not being listened to when saying something important. Also, the intense frustration of being misunderstood when the other person refuses or does not take the trouble to see things from your point of view. Equally, it is disturbing to realise that someone is saying one thing but meaning another. This is true not only in intimate relationships in personal life but also at work where the focus is on a job that has to be done.

These comments apply to people interacting with each other – the interpersonal world. There is also another world of communication within each person, the intrapsychic world. Comments such as 'He's his own worst enemy' or 'She's so critical of herself' suggest that reference to this internal communication is necessary to do justice to the rich complexity of human experience. It seems that people live simultaneously in the outside world and in an internal world of thought and feeling. For some personalities the interpersonal world is the most rewarding and is where they focus their attention. For others the intrapsychic world is the most real and offers the greatest rewards. Perhaps we are all seeking a balance between the two.

What is true about relations and communications between individuals and groups is also true about the internal thoughts and feelings of every human being. If the need to communicate with and explore other people is so strong why do so many people find it difficult and unrewarding? For some, relating to other people is considered risky or even dangerous and therefore the need for safety and security dominates the need to relate. Langs (1983) puts it thus:

> Communicative exchanges give substance to our lives; they are essential for survival and growth. We know that we require a sufficient amount of internal communication, as in private thoughts, fantasies and dreams to maintain our sanity. The need for expression is powerful in all human beings, although often it is compromised by strong needs for defence, non-communication, and withdrawal. Self-expression is important to all coping efforts and especially so in emotionally trying situations.

The focus of this book

Of all the ways of expressing thoughts and feelings – a political address, a dream, intimate words of affection, a poem or play, a scientific report, a painting, a piece of music – the focus of this book is on communication between individuals using the spoken word and associated elements. The communication can be between two individuals or a group of people and is assumed to be in a professional nursing setting,

for example, nurse/patient, nurse/nurse or nurse/doctor/manager.

This apparently simple process of one person talking to another is highly complex and subtle and needs to be analysed carefully if it is to be understood. Chapter 1 attempts to do this by defining the basic components of communication, outlining a specific model of communication and by building a fuller picture bit by bit to do justice to the complexity. Later chapters examine the influences which affect communication and how communication might be improved, as well as looking at communication in various settings.

THE BASIC COMPONENTS OF COMMUNICATION

Sender, message, receiver

The basic unit of communication is made up of a sender, a receiver and a message set within a particular context (Fig. 1.1). The sender intends to convey a particular message but may send much that is beyond direct awareness. The unconscious or hidden content of communication is an integral and important part of the whole. The message itself may be in line with conscious intentions or may be at considerable variance with them. Equally the receiver may register what was intended to be sent but often receives more as well, especially the unconscious component. The four variables interact, each contributing to the meaning of a communication.

In the example given in Box 1.1, the community psychiatric nurse might perceive how depressed the patient is in contradiction of the explicit message. A more naive observer might not pick up this message at all.

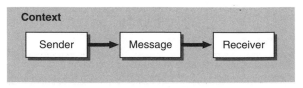

Fig 1.1 The basic components of communication

Box 1.1 The basic components of communication: example

Sender: patient
Message: I'm feeling just fine today
Receiver: community psychiatric nurse
Context: home visit

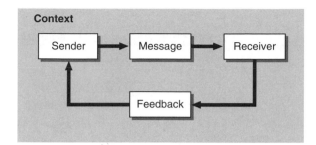

Fig 1.2 Basic components of communication with feedback

This simple diagram models a one-way communication only. Some people act as though there is no response to what they are communicating but the focus here is on two-way communication, where the receiver is actively involved in the process so that each person is modifying messages in the light of the other's response. Nevertheless, one-way communication is common even in the face-to-face situation between a doctor/nurse and nurse/patient. 'You should have been aware of the problems of this patient much sooner, nurse'. 'You're not to have anything to eat for 24 hours'.

Many who assent to two-way communication in theory do not practise it. Bradley & Edinberg (1990) give the following reasons why nurses may use one-way communication though they believe in a two-way model:

◆ The communicator controls one-way communication. Clearly, listening to a response makes demands on the nurse's capacity to adapt to the unexpected and she may feel more vulnerable or intimate with the patient as a result.
◆ One way communication can take place more easily whilst doing something else, e.g. whilst making the bed. Full attention on the receiver is not always necessary.
◆ Nurses feel under pressure to do lots of tasks. Two-way communication may take time away from other important aspects of patient care.

Menzies-Lyth (1960) studied the ways in which the social system of a hospital was organised to protect staff from being overwhelmed by the stress and anxiety generated by their jobs. Amongst these she noted the splitting up of the nurse/patient relationship by breaking down the total workload of a ward into lists of tasks each of which is allocated to a particular nurse. As a result the nurse has restricted contact with any one patient. Another technique she noted was that of depersonalisation, categorisation, and denial of the significance of the individual. These and other devices inhibit the development of a full person-to-person relationship between nurse and patient, with its consequent anxiety.

It is well worth considering other reasons from your own personal experience as to why one-way communication might be adopted and to remain alert to the consequences of one-way and two-way communication in practice.

With a feedback loop the first diagram now becomes a two-way communication (Fig. 1.2).

Basic principles of communication

Before developing a more elaborate model it may be helpful to consider four basic principles of communication based on the ideas of Watzlawick et al (1967) summarised in Box 1.2 and described in more detail here.

1. One cannot *not* communicate. All behaviour has a message of some sort so that as well as the more obvious carriers of messages like words or gestures, saying or doing nothing is itself a message. Not smiling is just as potent a message as smiling. Once a message has been sent it cannot be retracted. If a judge tells the jury to disregard the evidence given she cannot change the fact that the members have heard it. All communication is

---

Box 1.2 Watzlawick's four basic principles of communication

1. One cannot *not* communicate

2. Every communication has a content and relationship aspect such that the latter classifies the former and is therefore a metacommunication.

3. A series of communications can be viewed as an uninterrupted series of interchanges.

4. All communication relationships are either symmetrical or complementary depending on whether they are based on equality or inequality.

---

irreversible – as many a public figure has learned to her cost.

2. Every communication has a content and relationship aspect such that the latter classifies the former and is therefore a metacommunication. Any communication sequence has a message content and also has aspects which refer to the way in which the message is received. How communicators relate to each other is sometimes consciously controlled but is more commonly unconsciously controlled. Consider this exchange:

Patient: I don't want to take these pills.
Nurse: You must. Doctor says so.

The last comment is a communication about the communication (a metacommunication) and marks out clearly how the nurse sees her relationship to the patient – that of control. Chapter 3 looks in more detail at the effects of role and social context on communication.

3. A series of communications can be viewed as an uninterrupted series of interchanges. There is no clear beginning or ending to a series of interchanges: any communication between two individuals has a history and a future in itself and is affected by the totality of the past experiences of each individual. Hurtful past experiences can set up a pattern in which the person ignores the offender who then ignores the offended and thus the situation becomes

an unhelpful communication chain reaction. It is difficult to deal with this pattern when a patient's manner is habitually offensive.

4. All communication relationships are either symmetrical or complementary, depending on whether they are based on equality or inequality. With two equal partners, such as two close friends, the interaction is likely to be symmetrical. With a status or power differential between two people, such as a teacher and pupil or doctor and nurse, the complementary relationship (one 'superior' to the other) will affect any communication between them. In general, how any communication is interpreted depends on the relationship the sender has with the receiver. Again these issues of role, status and power are examined in more detail in Chapter 3.

With four basic principles of communication and a simple model in place it is now possible to develop a more complex model of communication which will form the basis of all further comments in this chapter.

A MODEL OF COMMUNICATION

Sending a message

The model illustrated in Figure 1.3 starts with the thoughts and feelings of the sender, i.e. the intrapsychic world, and acknowledges that these have to be encoded into some form of behaviour (the message) if they are to leave the internal domain and be communicated to another person (the receiver). The message of verbal and/or nonverbal signs and symbols needs to be carried by one means or another (the channels) on to one or more of the senses of the receiver so that the receiver can perceive it. From these sense data the receiver decodes and interprets the message and has thoughts and feelings as a result. These may or may not match the intended message of the sender. In any interaction the receiver is likely to have thoughts and feelings that she will encode in her own style and send back to the original sender. Thus the process of two-way communication proceeds.

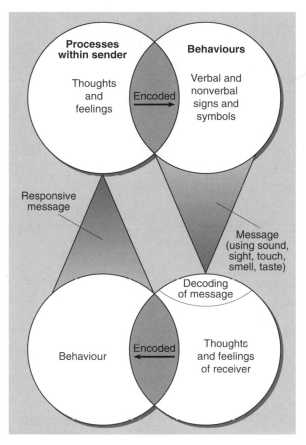

Fig 1.3 A model of communication

The message

Useful insights into the meaning of a word can often be gained by considering its derivation. The central element in the word 'message' is 'mess' which is still used in two distinct ways – to supply with meals and also to make dirty or untidy with extensions of bungling, interfering, disarranging or man-handling. Hence 'Don't mess with me!'

The derivation of the word message then contains both nurturing qualities and also the potential for confusing and hurting. Messages are indeed sent to create meaning but are also used defensively, to hide what is actually going on, to create confusion and attack relatedness. The work of Laing (1959) and others attempted to demonstrate that a patient's apparently bizarre symptoms

(labelled schizophrenic) could make sense if seen in the context of the original patterns of communication in the family which often had the quality of creating confusion and undermining relationships.

Perhaps the most compressed example of the subtlety of the mix of both aspects in a message, nurturing and hurtful, is in the 'double bind' (Bateson et al 1956). The victim of the double bind is caught inside contradictory statements so that she cannot do the right thing. Current pressure in the health service for quality care and for high turnover and efficiency may often be experienced by a nurse as contradictory. One message received may be clearly incompatible with the next message. Even more difficult to handle is the situation in which the overt message hides or disguises a covert contradictory message. 'Get the turnover rate up' but also implying, but not stating, 'and don't let the quality slip'. The nurse's dilemma is whether to base her action on the overt or the covert message. She is in a double bind, a 'Damned if you do, damned if you don't' situation. Thus messages are often not simple and can appear to be one thing when in fact they are another.

In contrast, the word 'communicate' has no negative overtones, implying only transmitting, making known and passing on of knowledge and information. Related words such as communion and community indicate the emphasis on qualities of sharing and fellowship. Thus communication has the positive and nurturing qualities of message but not the negative, messy ones.

Carriers of the message

In face-to-face communication a message is received through one or more of the five senses. The senses are the means by which a message originating in the external world is registered by the body and converted into internal experience. Messages are conveyed from one person to another through the senses in the following ways.

Language

A highly developed language is the supreme achievement of the human mind and body and is a development beyond the more primitive channels of communication discussed below. Language is necessary for the complex and abstract ideas needed for the intricacies of social organisation and culture. Consider the massive strides forward in civilisation that have taken place since a means was found to express spoken language in written form so that experience and knowledge could last beyond a human lifetime and be transmitted and received other than by face-to-face contact. Consider also the consequences socially and politically of being able to mass produce the written word.

The lexical content of a message, i.e. the words themselves, can only convey meaning if the receiver understands them. This is both obvious and frequently overlooked by senders of messages. Students often complain of teachers using abstract concepts and jargon to express meaning which 'goes over the head'. Nurses are sometimes asked after a doctor's visit to explain to patients what was said to them, i.e. to translate technical language into an intelligible form for those without such language. Part of becoming a nurse is being initiated into the concepts and ideas of a body of medical knowledge and to be able to use such language to communicate effectively to other professionals. It is also important to be able to keep the common touch.

Some people consciously (and unconsciously) use language to mystify, impress, dominate, humiliate and to give markers of their social position (see Chapter 3). This use of language is an example of sending multiple messages in which the surface meaning is secondary in importance to the disguised meaning. It is a common enough experience to be in the company of people whose use of technical language defines the boundaries of the group and excludes others. It is noticeable on some professional social occasions that there are forces around to unite groups who use a common language and to exclude others who may find the experience tiresome as a result. 'In-groups', like teenagers, need to keep language on the move with 'in-words' to mark the boundary between 'in' and 'out'.

Given that hearing is the sense that receives the lexical content in speech, a hearing loss is a severe impairment in face-to-face communication. Sign language of the deaf substitutes the sight channel for the hearing channel but is less symbolically rich. Counsellors of the deaf report how much more difficult it is to engage with the nuance and subtleties of feeling in their clients with hearing disabilities compared with clients who can hear. Also, sound carries in three-dimensional space – we can hear messages from any direction – whereas the eyes receive from the front only. However, the lexical content is only part of the transmitted message received by hearing; there is also nonverbal communication.

Paralinguistic features

These are the features of a spoken message that are not contained in the words alone, i.e. rhythm, pace, emphasis, intonation, pitch and tone of voice. A message such as 'I'll see you at 8 o'clock' can be a simple declaration or a question, depending on the intonation. Emphasis, pace and tone of voice can also make this into an authoritative bark or a seductive invitation.

Such features help in the interpretation of a message by giving the receiver clues about the sender's state of mind. Is she being angry, suspicious, sarcastic, serious, or funny? Loudness, stress and quality of voice encode some of these aspects of communication. The sentence 'She's really caring' can have quite different meanings depending on which word is stressed and contextual clues are likely to reinforce the intended meaning. Accent and dialect can show social class and regional origins and differences. It is impressive to note how much information passes between two people by these paralinguistic features from a single short utterance. In telephone conversations they are particularly important because visual clues from the other person are missing.

 Activity 1.1 An exercise in para-linguistic features

Take a simple sentence such as 'I'll see you in the library this afternoon' and, with a partner, experiment to see how many variations in meaning you can achieve simply by changing the way you say the words without actually altering any of them.

What can you deduce from this exercise?

Body language

These two words suggest that there is another channel for carrying meaning and communicating which does not use words at all. Body language has become a popular topic both in everyday conversation and in serious scientific studies of animal and human interaction. As every parent knows, a baby communicates effectively, if imprecisely, both its urgent needs and satisfactions through the use of gestures and nonverbal cries and noises. Each individual, through her own development, can be seen to recapitulate the human race's evolutionary past and this is true also of the development of communication – from gestures and actions, to meaningful grunts and noises, to more articulated sounds which eventually become the language. Visual signals also carry significant meaning and can replace, supplement or contradict a verbal message. Certain hand gestures, for example, are potent messages of affection or contempt and exist across many cultures in different forms. Car drivers, in particular, are subjected to enough of these gestures to be kept up to date on what is currently in vogue.

Dimbleby & Burton (1992) suggest that body language has several elements.

Gesture While people are speaking they gesture with their hands, some more than others. They provide useful information as experiments have shown in which people describe shapes or movements with or without using their hands (Argyle 1992). More subtle gestures include the steepling of the fingers to express confidence, and listeners often use head nods of different amplitude – small ones to show attention, larger and repeated ones to show agreement. Interestingly, gestures and speech are controlled by the same area of the brain and develop in children at about the same time.

Facial expressions Possibly because of their important survival value in infancy, subtle variations in smile or look are readily distinguished, especially those located around the eyes and mouth. Whether a listener is pleased, puzzled or annoyed can be detected by observing the eyes and mouth.

Gaze It follows that gaze is important in assessing nonverbal clues. Gaze is closely coordinated with speech: the speaker usually looks at the listener before making a major grammatical break and particularly before the end of utterances. Speakers often look away when they start to speak or are thinking about what they are saying.

Posture The way the body is held gives a general indication of confidence, attention, boredom, confrontation and other specific reactions. In Western culture people normally stand with their bodies slightly averted from each other when having a conversation to indicate polite friendliness or neutrality. Other cultures have different codes of behaviour and this can be disconcerting sometimes, leading to misunderstandings and even offence.

Body space and proximity People need a certain space around them to feel comfortable and this varies depending on age, sex and culture. Being squashed into a small space with other people in a lift or a crowded bus generally engenders feelings of awkwardness and discomfort with some relief when personal space is restored. Adults keep an arm's reach away from other people unless they know them reasonably well. It follows that the tensions involved for both parties when a nurse is physically handling and treating a patient are to be expected and need to be acknowledged.

Touch This tells a good deal about the nature of a relationship and the degree of friendliness between two people. It can also be used as a marker of status, the higher status person implying 'I can touch you but you should not touch me'. Touch is a potent carrier of messages as lovers, friends, relatives and victims of sexual harassment or abuse know. Clearly, different rules of behaviour exist in the medical world from those in everyday life. The traditional view has, perhaps unconsciously, taken heed of this potency by insisting on keeping an emotional distance between carer and patient. A gynaecological examination rarely has eye contact between doctor and patient during the process as if to suggest that to have eye contact as well as body contact would be emotionally too much. Conversely, those treatments which encourage a strong emotional attachment between carer and patient, e.g. psychotherapy, are those in which physical contact is normally regarded as unethical.

Dress The manner and presentation of dress, hair, jewellery and make-up say a lot about an individual's personality, role, job, status and mood. The use of a uniform is itself a strong statement that the role is more important than the individual. Nurses in some work settings may decide against wearing a uniform following discussions about the intended nature of the relationship between nurse and patient. Individuals in hospital hierarchies often code their position by different forms of dress.

Argyle found that when a stranger behaved in a friendly nonverbal style it created a much more friendly impression than the use of friendly words. He suggests several nonverbal signals that are effective in communicating a friendly attitude (see Box 1.3).

The visual, audible, verbal and nonverbal messages are normally presented together in face-to-face communication. Consistency is sought between the multiple channels with integration of all the information for the fullest picture. If, however, someone says 'I'm not angry' but bangs down her fist, the gesture perceived is often taken as the reliable source of information. Conflict and defensiveness are often expressed in such discrepant ways. In general, the verbal message is easier to manipulate and control than the nonverbal message because the first requires conscious processing whilst the latter is usually unconscious. A nurse may intuitively know that a patient is distressed even though the patient has just said 'I'm all right' because nonverbal messages have been sent and received in clear contradiction of the words uttered. In counselling and psychotherapy a client will frequently tell a grim story with either no emotional tone or with a smile. This discrepancy indicates that the feeling content of the message is difficult to express or 'face'.

Box 1.3 The nonverbal signals of a friendly attitude (from Argyle 1992)	
Proximity:	closer, lean forward if seated
Orientation:	more direct, but side to side for some situations
Gaze:	more gaze and mutual gaze
Facial expression:	more smiling
Gestures:	head nods, lively movements
Posture:	open arms stretched towards each other rather than arms on hips or folded
Touch:	more touch in an appropriate manner
Tone of voice:	higher pitch, upward contour, pure tone
Verbal contents:	more self-disclosure

THE SENDER AND RECEIVER

The model of communication given earlier makes a clear distinction between processes happening within a person (essentially unobservable) and behaviour that is emitted by a person (public and observable). The emitted behaviour is the content and channel of the message being sent between sender and receiver. Consideration is now given to how a person's behaviour (external world – interpersonal) is linked to her experience of thoughts and feelings (internal world – intrapsychic). The relationship between behaviour and experience is subtle and far-reaching and some of the ideas about the inner world of the person must be explored.

The personal internal world

Psychodynamic theory addresses the intrapsychic world of the person and formulates concepts and ideas to describe and explain it. The first idea is that the forces which shape any human life belong not only to the present – the here and now – but also in the past, especially the distant past, i.e. the early life of childhood and even babyhood. A second idea is that human behaviour is best explained in terms of mental processes that are not only unobservable to outsiders but that are also to a large extent unknowable to the individual, i.e. they are unconscious. This latter idea provides rich insights into the subtleties and difficulties of human communication. It enables common experiences in communication to be addressed, for example:

◆ Understanding the words that someone has said but also having a vague yet strong intuition that there is another unsaid message, often of an emotional sort. Feelings of confusion, bewilderment and unease are not uncommon in such circumstances.

◆ The way in which individuals have their own code of expression, especially when strong negative emotions are aroused. A person treated appallingly by a colleague might say 'It wasn't a very nice thing to do'. Such idiosyncrasies of expression need to be understood and acknowledged if the full force of a communication is to be appreciated.

◆ Receiving attacks on one's capacity to communicate and have peace of mind especially from patients who are, either temporarily or chronically, emotionally disturbed. Segal (1991) says that her own observations have shown how clearly a sense of one's own goodness and worth seems to depend on physical health so it is not surprising that people are often emotionally disturbed when they become patients – a fact which is often denied by health professionals.

Some light can be thrown on such common everyday experiences by focusing on the remarkable ability of the human mind to express itself simultaneously on two distinct and yet related levels of meaning. People often express themselves in a single, direct way without any hint of a second meaning. At other times there is a shift to a more complex way of functioning in which encoded messages are generated that have both a surface meaning and a disguised meaning (see Fig. 1.4).

The shift from one form of expression to the other can be quite conscious. One thing is often said which deliberately means something else. If, however, circumstances are highly emotionally

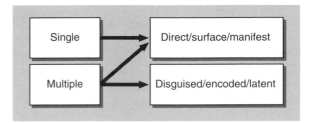

Fig 1.4 Single and multiple levels of communication

charged, either internally or in the outside world, then the shift from one form of expression to the other is beyond conscious control and multiple level messages are deployed unconsciously.

Taken together, a more complex picture of communication emerges in which a person's inner world – the intrapsychic domain – is interacting with any interpersonal messages that are being exchanged. It is because of this interaction that each person has enormous resources for subtle and complex communication with others. It is these resources that can keep friendships and other intimate relationships alive for a lifetime.

To summarise, it is part of normal human development to:

◆ give surface messages with direct and simple meaning;
◆ consciously encode a secondary message below the surface message where indirectness is intended; and
◆ unconsciously deal with difficult emotional situations by encoding messages in disguised form without being aware of doing so.

These three modes of communication from everyday life can now be examined in more detail together with a fourth, commonly known as 'dumping' (Box 1.4).

Direct surface messages

Direct surface messages are vital for survival and depend on logic and reason for their content and form. Many human transactions in the medical world depend on reliable information being

---

Box 1.4 Four modes of communication

1. Surface messages with direct and simple meaning.
2. Consciously encoded messages which contain a secondary message below the surface.
3. Unconsciously encoded messages in which feelings are unconsciously disguised to protect the individual from a disturbing experience/emotion.
4. 'Dumping' whereby an individual gets rid of disturbing experiences/emotions by dumping them on to someone else.

Box 1.5 Consciously encoded messages: an example

Sister: What with staff shortages and a holiday coming up I don't know how we are going to cope.
Nurse: I've already worked two double shifts this week.
Sister: I'll be on duty throughout the Bank Holiday.
Nurse: Yes, I know. I covered for Jenny the other day when she was off sick.

---

transmitted from one person to another without ambiguity or distortion. The safe treatment of a patient is built upon such communication. 'Give this patient 10 milligrams twice a day' and 'Pass me the spatula' are examples of the common occurrence of medical communication that makes any treatment possible. Meaning is clear and the use of language, given a common understanding by sender and receiver of vocabulary and grammar, is limited to dealing with direct surface messages. It is disturbing to the receiver in these circumstances not to understand what is being said, either at the lexical level (not knowing the meaning of a word) or by an unfamiliar use of intonation, accent or dialect. Difficulties are located in the message itself, not in the decoding of the sender's intention. Context has the power to change the surface meaning of even the simplest message. 'I'll kill you if you do that' will be interpreted differently when said with a threatening knife or during a playful episode.

Surface messages have utility, hence their importance, but little else. Conversation in the interpersonal realm is rather bleak if it is made up of surface messages only because all is clear – there is no allusion or implication to stimulate the imagination. In the TV series Star Trek, Mr Spock is infuriating at times to Captain Kirk because of the computer-like logic of his conversation.

Conscious encoding

If the surface message is part of a multiple level message then, to be effective, it must not only be understood on its own terms but also point to a hidden meaning suitably encoded and disguised. The power of great poems, plays or novels stems from their capacity to engage imaginatively at the surface level but also to point to mysterious underlying levels of coded messages that are sensed rather than understood.

In everyday life, deliberate encoding is often employed when tact, consideration and sensitivity are desirable and when a direct message is inadvisable. Painful messages are often expressed through such encoding and the main function of this type of message is to soften the blow, to take advantage of all the means available whereby something is better not fully said. The medical world is full of situations in which painful messages have to be given to patients or their relatives and yet there seems some reluctance to examine, in human terms, the process of giving such a message (Kubler-Ross 1970).

Box 1.5 shows an everyday conversation between hospital staff in which both parties consciously encode their messages in the hope of achieving desired results. The sister makes two statements of fact which carry an uncomfortable message for the nurse who struggles to defend herself from the implications using equally encoded messages.

People vary in their responsiveness to encoded messages. The underlying raw message can be avoided by pretending it does not exist. This is often an attempt to frustrate the sender of the encoded communication, attack the intended meanings and preclude any further creative communication along the hidden lines. Another approach is to confront the disguise and to state the 'unsaid' message directly. This is likely to be received as tactless because such a strategy does not respect the need for the encoding in the first place. Perhaps the most common coping method is to register the hidden meaning and to make an appropriate encoded response in return as the nurse does in the example in Box 1.5.

Activity 1.2 An exercise in conscious encoding

Think of situations in which your superior gave you a derivative encoded message together with a surface message. How did you respond? How would you give such a message if the roles were reversed?

Unconscious encoding

This is far too big a subject to be treated in anything but an outline form here. Individuals learn from childhood to protect themselves from dangerous emotions by unconsciously avoiding them and communicating in messages distant from the threatening feelings yet derived from them. A patient may be full of bluster and bravado and be quite unaware that she is afraid.

Activity 1.3 An exercise in unconscious encoding

Think of examples of ways in which patients have unconsciously disguised their feelings in order to protect themselves from disturbing experiences.

How have you been able to relate the inferences from their behaviour to the hidden underlying message?

Such unconscious encoding is universal and it is useful for health professionals to be aware of the general indicators which point to hidden, derivative messages from patients. Considerable caution needs to be applied when trying to understand unconscious messages: it is easy to over-interpret and to misread a straightforward communication. It is also inevitable that the receiver will project personal issues into the communication, at least to some extent, and so contaminate the sender's message. Conversely, there is also the danger that a communication will be taken at face value when, in reality, an important encoded message is being sent which is consequently missed.

There are many clues to suggest someone is sending an encoded message:

◆ The message may not seem entirely logical, realistic or complete. Clearly many factors have to be considered in order to reach this conclusion – the wider context, the trigger for the communication – and such evaluation should be tentative and should seek validation from other sources.

◆ There may be contradictions in the communication flow so that one element does not fit in with the general theme(s) and this is noticed by the receiver.

◆ There may be a discrepancy between how the sender intended the message to be received and understood and how it is actually received. This is the area that most needs external validation if the personal bias of the receiver is not to dominate the interpretation.

◆ The sender may make inexplicable errors, for example, misperceptions, lapses of memory, behaviour that seems out of keeping with conscious thoughts and intentions, slips of the tongue.

◆ Strong feelings and highly emotional situations are likely to evoke encoded messages with important hidden meanings. This is true where conflict and anxiety are strongly present and also where there is a sense of danger or mistrust.

◆ The presence of psychosomatic symptoms – phobias, obsessions, anxiety – is another clue to emotional disturbance and the presence of hidden messages.

These indicators of the presence of unconscious encoding of messages need to be assessed with caution. However, given that the health care context is likely to foster the use of messages with important encoded meanings, it can help genuine communication considerably if health professionals are aware of this dimension to ordinary human contact.

Dumping

Any attempt to define communication would be incomplete without addressing a familiar experience in human interaction, commonly known as dumping. When dumping, individuals are not concerned with communicating meaning but with getting rid of feelings or something disturbing within themselves – an evacuation process.

The goal of the dumper is either to discharge internal discomfort by creating a comparable disturbance in the receiver (an unconscious wish 'I'll make you feel as bad as I do'), or to get the receiver to incorporate the disturbance to see how she deals with it ('I'll put my bad feelings into you and see how you cope with it'). Nurses frequently report experiences with patients that make them feel agitated and upset. The patient offloads disturbing feelings on to the nurse who subsequently feels 'dumped' into and exploited as if she is carrying the discomfort that was originally with the patient.

For some individuals the desire to rid themselves of inner disturbance goes alongside a desire to understand their inner and interpersonal struggles. Once dumping is over they can take part in a quieter form of meaningful communication and explore underlying issues. There are others who want only to get rid of what disturbs them and to upset the receiver. They are neither interested in

understanding what they are doing and why, nor are they concerned for the effect which the dumping may have on the receiver.

Dumping is a maladaptive means of communicating. It is focused on action and discharge rather than reflection and creates alienation and antagonism. It is not uncommon for a known dumper, whether patient or colleague, to clear the social space of listeners as soon as she appears! Dumping can bring no lasting comfort to the dumper because this method of communicating cannot enhance growth, learning or reflection. Dumpers are prisoners of their communication style and endlessly repeat the dumping process in a vain attempt to secure relief from internal tension.

Finally, it is important to recognise our own dumping tendencies and to manage and contain them from our own internal resources. In addition, the ability to recognise dumping tendencies in others can foster effective communicative reactions

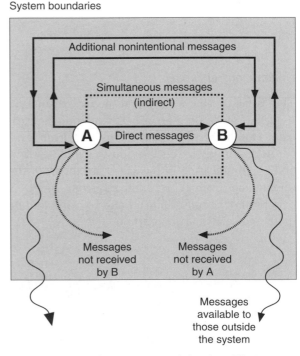

System boundaries

Fig 1.5 A model of communication (taken from Ellis & McClintock 1990)

within ourselves, which otherwise would lead to communicative misunderstanding and alienation.

A final model of communication

We are now in a position to represent some of this complexity in a final diagram (see Fig. 1.5).

This takes account of the fact that there is probably an enormous number of messages flowing between those involved in one-to-one communication: some messages never get through to the receiver; some are disregarded even when they do get through; and some messages are perceived only by those outside the interaction.

CONCLUSION

This chapter has taken a broad look at the nature of face-to-face human communication: direct, indirect, conscious, unconscious and dumping. Like so many other aspects of human life, communication becomes more complicated the closer it is examined and our definition of the word should now be much broader than might have been expected at the outset. In the next chapter we look closely at the person in communication, i.e. the sender and receiver of messages, and use the theoretical ideas of psychologists to further develop our view of human communication.

REFERENCES

Argyle M 1992 The social psychology of everyday life. Routledge, London

Bateson G, Jackson DD, Haley J, Weakland J 1956 Toward a theory of schizophrenia. Behavioural Science 1: 251

Bradley JC, Edinberg MA 1990 Communication in the nursing context, 3rd edn. Appleton and Lange, Connecticut

Dimbleby R, Burton G 1992 More than words: an introduction to communication, 2nd edn. Routledge, London

Ellis R, McClintock A 1990 If you take my meaning. Arnold, London

Kubler-Ross E 1970 On death and dying. Tavistock/Routledge, London

Laing RD 1959 The divided self. Tavistock, London

Langs R 1983 Unconscious communication in everyday life. Jason Aronson, New York

Menzies-Lyth I 1988 The functioning of social systems as a defence against anxiety. In: Menzies-Lyth I (ed) Containing anxiety in institutions – Selected essays. Free Association Books, London

Segal J 1991 The use of the concept of unconscious phantasy in understanding reactions to chronic illness. In: Counselling. The Journal of the British Association for Counselling 2(4)

Watzlawick P, Beavin J, Jackson D 1967 Pragmatics of human communication. Norton, New York

FURTHER READING

Berryman J 1987 Psychology and you. Methuen, London

Burton G, Dimbleby R 1988 Between ourselves. Arnold, London

Cooper CL 1986 Improving interpersonal relations. Wildwood House, Aldershot

Hein EC 1980 Communication in nursing practice, 2nd edn. Little, Brown, Boston

Morrison P, Burnard P 1991 Caring and communicating. Macmillan, London

Wainwright GR 1985 Body language. Hodder and Stoughton, Kent

2

The person in communication

Roger Ellis   Bob Gates

INTRODUCTION

The previous chapter looked at the nature of communication and compiled a complex picture based on the simple definition of sender, message, and receiver. We emphasised the message, its nature, and its capacity to have single and multiple meanings and the ways in which it could be sent and received. In this chapter we focus on the sender and receiver, i.e. on the persons who are communicating. To understand the meaning of a message, assumptions are necessarily made about the person who sent it. This is true not only of an individual person but also of people in general.

The link between communication and assumptions about people can be frequently observed. Children are often treated as if they do not understand what is happening around them when they quite clearly do. People with a physical disability often complain about bizarre assumptions made of them, for example, that they are deaf or unintelligent. The bedside communication between a doctor and a nurse in a hospital situation might reveal to the patient their assumptions about the role of a sick person. The power of role along with context to determine the nature of communication is examined in more detail in Chapter 3.

In order to examine what these general underlying assumptions might be and in order to assess alternatives, we need first to have some knowledge of the theory of human nature. People observe other people and develop theories about why others behave as they do and how they are different. For professional carers it is necessary to have some means of predicting how people are going to behave in general even if each is treated as an individual. Effective caring practice is built on coherent theory, which is itself built on basic assumptions. Actions need to be grounded in theory if they are not to be random and incoherent. For practice to be more effective, we need to make explicit the underlying assumptions and theory which otherwise remain implicit and hidden.

PSYCHODYNAMIC, BEHAVIOURIST AND HUMANISTIC THEORY

There are three theoretical approaches to the person in communication, which are commonly used in a nursing context – the psychodynamic, the behaviourist and the humanistic theories. Each has arisen in a particular context for a particular purpose and each makes a significant contribution to an understanding of the complexity of human nature. In this chapter we concentrate on the different basic concepts, principles, assumptions and applicability of each theory. Individuals will then be in a position to compare their own personal theory-making with that of other specialists in the field, and potentially gain new insights into communication with others.

What divides the theorists?

There are six basic issues which divide theorists (Pervin 1993) and which reflect the personal life experiences of the theorists as well as the social and scientific trends current at the time of their work (see Box 2.1). The way in which these issues are addressed affects the way in which a person is viewed and which aspects of human functioning are chosen for emphasis and investigation.

The philosophical view

People rarely need to articulate to each other the values and beliefs that underlie their view of the world. Any coherent theory of the person is built upon a philosophical view concerning human nature. One theory emphasises instinctive forces,

> **Box 2.1** Six basic issues to divide theorists (Pervin 1993)
>
> 1. The philosophical view of the person.
> 2. The relation between internal (personal) and external (situational) influences in determining behaviour.
> 3. The concept of the self and how to account for organised functioning.
> 4. The role of varying states of awareness.
> 5. The relationships between feeling, thought and behaviour.
> 6. The role of the past, present and future in governing behaviour.

another social factors. Are people driven or are they free? Rational or compulsively irrational? Self-seeking or capable of altruism? Spiritual or biological beings? These issues and many others have been debated throughout history and are at the root of any major shift in the perception and treatment of patients receiving medical care.

When seeking to understand a philosophical model it is useful to consider its philosophical base. The model that best suits an individual will be influenced by personal factors, life experiences, culture and by the spirit of the times, just as the original proponents of each model were so influenced. The psychodynamic model – with its origins in Freud's ideas – views the person as a product of early experiences. Skinner's (1938) behaviourist view believes behaviour is a response to the environment and the feedback received from it. Carl Rogers' (1970) humanistic, or person-centred view is that each individual is a self-actualising organism which has a basically positive drive towards health and happiness.

Internal and external forces

A second and related issue is whether the causes of behaviour are inside a person or outside in the environment. The extreme views are easy to recognise. Freud believes unknown internal forces within the unconscious control human beings, whereas Skinner suggests that a person does not act upon the world, the world acts upon him, i.e. environmental forces control him. To a certain extent all views are interactive but it is worth asking whether the focus of any one view is on internal, personal factors or on external, environmental factors.

The concept of self

To be a distinct person is to have some coherent, consistent pattern and organisation of thought, feeling and behaviour. To account for this aspect of human functioning the concept of self has been used. Awareness of self is an important part of experience. The way individuals feel about themselves affects their outlook on the world and their behaviour towards others. Theorists differ considerably in their use of the self. Rogers makes it the central integrating concept as the person seeks to make the self and experience congruent with each other. Skinner in principle avoids the very notion of self as a vague, romantic and fanciful idea.

Awareness and consciousness

It is generally recognised by psychologists that the potential exists for different states of consciousness in human experience. Nevertheless, there is strong disagreement as to whether the concept of the unconscious is useful or necessary to explain the diverse phenomena of experience. How are dreams accounted for? Can people give an accurate account of themselves or are large parts of their thoughts, feelings and behaviour outside their awareness? The answers to these and other questions determine how people communicate and how they interpret what is said. If a nurse asks a patient how he is feeling does she take the answer to be the truth of the matter or are other factors to be taken into account?

Thoughts, feelings and behaviour

Theorists differ in the relative weight they give to each of these areas of functioning. From the psychodynamic view all behaviour is a product of

thought and feeling. Behaviourists focus on overt behaviour and reject any investigation of internal processes. Other theorists argue that thoughts are primary and cause both feelings and behaviour. Still others argue that emotions are primary and can direct thought and behaviour. Although there is a growing acceptance that all three aspects influence each other, the relative emphasis of one over the others distinguishes one model of the person from another.

The past, present and future

Is behaviour determined by the past or by expectations of the future, or solely by factors in the present? This is yet another issue that divides theorists. The distinguishing feature in each of the different theories is how the links between all three – past, present and future – are conceptualised. If people are viewed as being determined by their past with little hope for change they are unlikely to be treated differently, with a more optimistic view of the future. A nurse's whole basis for communication with a patient is built on his view of the relation between the present state of affairs and a prospective future. Having examined the basic issues that divide theorists, the three models can now be examined in more detail.

THE PSYCHODYNAMIC MODEL

The psychodynamic understanding of the person is derived from the work of Sigmund Freud. His theories and techniques of psychoanalysis have provided a rich source of ideas that many others have since developed and modified. This has given rise to a vast and complex literature involving many different schools of thought, which can be confusing and overwhelming to a new reader.

The word 'psychodynamic' is a useful one because it refers not to one theory only but to the many theories that owe their origins to the pioneering work of Freud. The two parts to the word offer some insight into the focus of the model. 'Psyche' is sometimes understood as mind but is best seen as referring to the whole of a person's

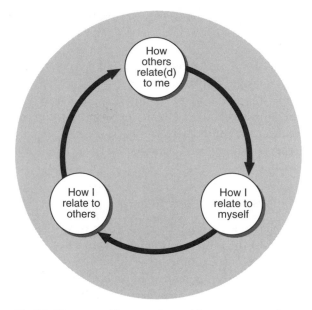

Fig 2.1 The external becomes internal becomes external

1. Each individual is the product and author of his own particular history: how he is now is a direct consequence of his earliest experiences with others and his environment. Subsequent experience confirms or modifies that early experience, for better or worse. He is not, however, passive in his history, but contributes to its shape.

2. He lives simultaneously in his external and internal worlds: the former he is mostly aware of, but the latter is primarily unconscious. The unconscious, internal world is energetic and substantially determines his feelings and actions in the external world.

3. All behaviour, no matter how apparently irrational and senseless, is logical and purposeful according to some personal system.

4. Chronological growth is inexorable, but emotional growth is beset by anxieties and detoured by defences and so doesn't always keep pace. Emotional disturbance is likely to be caused by some outdated and no longer appropriate motivation, decision (defence) or wish.

inner world of feelings, thoughts and experiences. Older words such as soul and spirit need to be added to do justice to the word 'psyche'. 'Dynamic' refers to the view that the psyche is seen as active and not static, not only relating to other people but also active within itself, relating to itself. Reflection on experience and the way we describe experience, e.g. 'I just did it. I don't know why. I feel so cross with myself' often reveals a person's internal relationships which are full of feeling and are not necessarily linked to other people at all. Thus the dynamic is both internal and external and the word 'psychodynamic' applies to the internal world of experience which in turn affects the external world. The way in which we relate to ourselves – with compassion, hatred, fear or envy – is expressed outside in the way we relate to others. Hence our style of communicating with others is derived from our communication with ourselves (see Fig. 2.1).

Object Relations theory

Freud's original theory emphasised the instinctive drives of the individual alone. Object Relations theory, a development from Freud, puts centre stage the need of human beings to relate to each other and shows how early relationships become internalised and repeated in the ways in which a person relates to himself and others. The term 'object' is somewhat confusing initially because it refers usually to persons and relationships rather than things. The basic assumptions of the psychodynamic Object Relations model of the person are concisely given by Noonan (1983) in Box 2.2 and are briefly described below.

Product and author

Individuals are generally viewed as products of the environment and the time and place in history.

People develop conceptions about themselves, about whether they are lovable, clever and good-looking, or unlovable, stupid and ugly. These perceptions enable the person to make sense of the world and make it predictable. An expectation of being rejected will affect the interaction with the next unfamiliar person we meet. This tendency will result in the achievement of the 'self-fulfilling prophecy'.

Harder to accept is the fact that these adult feelings and behaviours have roots in the much earlier experiences of childhood and infancy. Patterns of relating to our earliest figures, usually parents, are internalised resulting in an internal world that is dominated by feelings of anxiety and fear, or of confidence and worth. These early experiences are beyond normal memory, leaving unconscious constructions and expectations about later life. Conscious and deliberate interpretations are made about what is happening in the present and these factors actively contribute to shaping behaviour. Individuals are both product and author of their own history.

Those in the medical profession often have to live with the tension of ambivalent feelings towards a patient. Knowing that to some extent patients are victims of circumstances arouses a desire to help and serve the patient's best interests by understanding and compassion. However, it is common to see quite clearly how much a patient is contributing to his present condition, sometimes consciously but often quite unconsciously. It is difficult for a patient to hold both 'product and author' in mind and to take some appropriate responsibility for his present condition. It is also difficult for carers when the patient will not take responsibility and will not cooperate. The examples in Box 2.3 give illustrations of this tension.

External and internal worlds

The second assumption makes the reality of the unconscious mind a centrepiece. It can safely be said that the unraveling of the workings of the unconscious was one of Freud's major contributions to understanding the human person. All sorts of things

---

Box 2.3 Patients being products and authors

One of the recent debates in medicine has been centred on whether a doctor is justified in refusing to operate on patients with heart conditions who refuse to stop smoking. The moral dilemma rests on whether the doctor is obliged to treat the patient without his cooperation even though the treatment may be less effective as a result or whether the doctor should choose patients who do accept responsibility for their condition and are prepared to act accordingly.

The issues of suicide and euthanasia involve allied considerations of responsibility.

---

can be unconscious: drives, wishes, conflicts, fears, values, aims, defences, images of people and the self, and relationships.

Psychodynamic theorists such as Klein (1963) have suggested that unconscious phantasy underlies all thinking and feeling, not just the feelings of conscious awareness. Such phantasy begins very early in childhood and is primarily concerned with bodily processes and relating to others. It becomes more and more symbolic and elaborate during growth and development but it never loses its primitive roots in infancy. Phantasies about being abandoned, lost or heroically saved, for example, seem to exist independently of whether any of these things actually happened in reality. They appear to be products of the mind rather than of direct experience even though such events do also actually happen.

This internal world constantly interacts with the external one and people live simultaneously in both. When both worlds are in harmony there are no problems in living. It is when the conscious and unconscious wishes and aims differ that conflict and confusion are experienced. If the boundary between the two worlds becomes blurred it is possible to misconstrue people and events in potentially disastrous ways. The unconscious internal world is energetic because of its origins in infancy and when it surfaces it does so with the force of infantile feeling that can be highly disturbing. Box 2.4 gives examples of these points.

All behaviour is logical

The third assumption asserts that all behaviour has meaning if looked for. What appears to be bizarre behaviour in the present is usually derived from the demands of the unconscious breaking through the defence structure, from patterns of long ago in childhood, or as a result of living in a permanently defensive way. At some time in the past coping strategies may have been necessary and comforting but are now anachronistic. The present behaviour derived from them now seems senseless or maladaptive but if the whole historic picture were to be known it would make sense. The term defence is used to refer to the ways in which the human psyche has evolved to protect itself from the feelings of anxiety that inevitably arise from unconscious forces. Box 2.5 gives a list of common defence mechanisms.

Such defence mechanisms have a positive aspect in that they help the individual control and understand emotional experiences. When defences are down the person may be unable to function and feel overwhelmingly vulnerable. Defence mechanisms, however, also have a negative aspect when they are so strong that they make it difficult to act spontaneously or with trust. Thus potentially rewarding experiences may be inaccessible to the over-defensive person.

Box 2.4 Intrusion of the unconscious into conscious life

Patients often relate to nurses in a way that is not typical of adult functioning but reveals early emotional attachments. The 'good' nurse is one who cares and to care is to do all that the patient requests. A 'bad' nurse is one who is not absolutely devoted to the wellbeing of the patient and who has to deal with others too. Attitudes to different nurses often have this split quality in which one can do no wrong and another can do no right. Klein suggests that this is the way in which babies relate to their mothers – mother is either all good or all bad – and in the case below this is the way the patient is relating unconsciously to the nurses.

Helen has one patient on her ward, Mrs A, who relates to her in highly unpredictable ways. She never knows what is awaiting her when she comes on duty. On one occasion Mrs A goes on at length about how wonderful Helen is and what an ideal nurse she makes. At another, Helen is attacked and upbraided for her unfeeling neglect of Mrs A who seems mortally wounded if Helen has to attend to someone else. Helen finds these violent swings of mood difficult to deal with and tends to reduce contact with Mrs A to a minimum.

Klein suggests that such ruthless use of the nurse as either an ideal object or a completely bad object is typical of early patterns of relating and can be assumed to be unconscious in Mrs A.

Box 2.5 Common defence mechanisms

1. Repression: Unconscious exclusion of memories, feelings, etc. from awareness in order to prevent anxiety or guilt.

2. Denial: protecting oneself from painful reality by a refusal to recognise anxiety-provoking elements.

3. Displacement: transferring feelings or actions from their original target to another object that arouses less anxiety.

4. Reaction formation: disguising unconscious motivation by behaving in the opposite way.

5. Projection: attributing one's own (undesirable) traits to other people or agencies.

6. Intellectualisation: masking anxiety-arousing feelings by discussing them in a detached, intellectual manner.

7. Rationalisation: devising apparently rational, socially approved reasons for one's behaviour.

Emotional development

The fourth assumption points to the fact that the growth linked to the passage of time, such as physical development and ageing, has a given and irreversible quality about it. Emotional development on the other hand is not linear or steady and has many a detour and reversal. The term 'fixation' is applied if emotional development stops altogether and 'regression' if there is a reversion to an earlier state or way of functioning. Patients frequently show regressive behaviour, i.e. they act and feel as though they were much younger, especially when they are stressed, as they often are when ill. Being helpless and dependent may make the strongest of patients feel so anxious that he may well regress to a more infantile state and is then likely to feel the other anxieties of that stage, such as unrealistic fears of danger or abandonment.

The psychodynamic model of the person uses many concepts that have found their way into everyday language but which are here used in a more technical and restricted way, e.g. phantasy, defence and regression. Another important concept is transference. This is the process by which one person unconsciously relates to another in present circumstances in ways that are derived from the past. A nurse, for example, might react to a doctor as if he were his mother. He may know that the doctor is not at all like his mother but nevertheless find himself having familiar feelings whenever the doctor talks to or looks at him. See Box 2.6 for an illustration.

Application and limitation

The psychodynamic concepts and assumptions outlined here interrelate to give a coherent picture of the person. Such a view is helpful when communication with or from others has a component of indirectness, of something alluded to but not made explicit, as outlined in Chapter 1. When things are straightforward there is no need to resort to the concepts of the unconscious to help explain behaviour. It is worth remembering that ill or stressed patients are likely to behave in ways quite untypical of their normal behaviour and it is useful to have some ideas available that can potentially make sense of what is happening.

Although it can help to be aware of psychic mechanisms in communication with others, a deeper

---

Box 2.6 Illustration of transference at work

Diane, the eldest of four children, remembers her childhood as one in which her mother was never quite available for her emotionally. She always seemed to be busy with something or somebody else who Diane felt was more important than she was. Diane had an unconscious phantasy that if only she could do more for her mother and be a good little helper and carer she would receive the attention from her mother that she longed for.

From an early age, Diane had chosen nursing as her career. She threw herself into her training and her job and all was well for a while. Then she began to feel that other people's needs were like demands that she could not refuse and therefore resented and for which Diane felt she never received adequate recognition. A vicious circle developed in which Diane became more and more attentive and more and more tired and resentful. It was after a considerable period of guilt and depressive feelings that Diane realised painfully that her motives for coming into nursing had more to do with her unresolved relationship with her mother than with actually caring for the wellbeing of patients. She had transferred into the work situation, initially quite unconsciously, patterns of behaving and relating from her early childhood.

This is an example of what Bowlby (1979) has called 'compulsive care-giving' and what Malan (1979) has called the 'helping profession syndrome'. The person compulsively gives to others what he would like to have for himself which, as Malan notes, leads to 'a severe deficit in the emotional balance of payments'.

exploration with a patient into his feelings and the meaning of his behaviour is likely to need a great deal of time and skill. This type of help is more the remit of counselling and psychotherapy. Nevertheless, given that treatment of illness and communication with patients is now seen to involve a relationship between patient and carer, it is not surprising that some writers in the field (e.g. Balint 1964) suggest that an understanding of psychodynamic processes is required to effectively treat a person's entire illness rather than the disease or symptoms alone.

It is perhaps now possible for the reader to reexamine the six issues that divide theorists (see Box 2.1) and to identify where the psychodynamic model stands relative to each.

BEHAVIOURISM

At the turn of the last century a group of psychologists became dissatisfied with the psychodynamic approach to the explanation and understanding of the person and developed a new school of psychology known as behaviourism. Pivotal to this perspective was the theory that all behaviour rested on learnt responses to given stimuli, often referred to as associative, connectionist or behavioural theory. This relationship between a stimulus and a response by an organism is accounted for by an understanding of both classical and operant conditioning.

The behavioural model

The behavioural perspective of understanding the person is grounded in early psychological research into the nature of learning. This approach to understanding learning was first described by a neurophysiologist called Pavlov who, in 1902, described a relationship between unconditioned responses and unconditioned stimuli. The response was called unconditioned because it was reflexive in nature, implying that it was an integral component of the organism's repertoire of behaviour. The most

famous example of this was his description of the response of salivation by a dog to the presence of food. In a series of experiments on dogs Pavlov found that if an unconditioned stimulus (food) was paired with a conditioned stimulus (bell) then it would be possible to elicit a conditioned response. This is demonstrated in Figure 2.2 as occurring in three stages. In Stage 1, the unconditioned stimulus (the food) causes the dog to respond by salivating. If this unconditioned response (Stage 2) is paired for a sufficient period of time with a conditioned stimulus (the bell) then eventually the response of salivation can be obtained by using the conditioned stimulus alone. That is, the response becomes conditioned to the sound of the bell.

The work of Pavlov was extremely important at the turn of the last century in shaping the thinking of the emerging group of American psychologists now referred to as behaviourists. Of these psychologists, John Watson became credited as the founder of behaviourism. He believed that in order for psychology to become a science, its data had to be objective and measurable. He was not concerned with introspective, hypothetical causes of behaviour but with public, observable and measurable causes. Watson argued that behaviour was the direct result of conditioning. He believed this

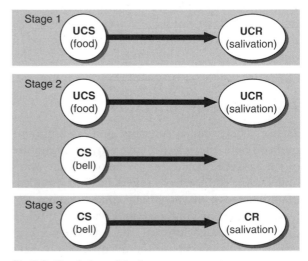

Fig 2.2 Classical conditioning

conditioning emanated from the environment in which the organism was located and that this environment would shape an organism's behaviour by reinforcing specific behaviours.

He further believed that simple chains of stimulus/response connections formed into longer, more complex strings of behaviour. These strings of behaviour, he argued, explained how a person thought and what motivated him. In addition, they accounted for personality, emotion, learning and remembering. The strength of such beliefs was clearly articulated by Watson (1924) when he said:

> *Give me a dozen healthy infants, well-formed, and my own specified world to bring them up in and I'll guarantee to take any one at random and train him to become any kind of specialist I might select – lawyer, artist, merchant, chief and yes even a beggar man and thief, regardless of his talents, penchants, abilities, vocations, and race of his ancestors. (Watson 1924)*

This underlying assumption can be seen to be in complete contrast to the psychodynamic approach described earlier in this chapter. From this early work on behaviourism emerged, amongst others, the work of Skinner (1938). His work, known as operant conditioning, latterly became known as behaviour modification. Skinner's contribution in this area is important because he was the first psychologist to point to the clinical and social relevance of operant conditioning (Bellack et al 1982). The next section provides examples of the application of behaviourism, which has been used as a therapeutic strategy to deal with psychological disorder and to improve or develop communication.

Operant conditioning

Operant conditioning suggests that when an organism makes a connection between a stimulus, the elicited response and the subsequent rewards or punishment, then its behaviour is reinforced either negatively or positively (see Fig. 2.3).

Behaviourists believe that if behaviour is reinforced positively then the incidence of that behaviour will increase. Conversely, if a behaviour is negatively reinforced the incidence of that behaviour will decrease. The essential difference between operant and classical conditioning is that in the latter the behaviour is a part of the animal's repertoire of behaviour. For example, salivation is a naturally occurring response of some organisms to food which can become conditioned by the repeated pairing of a conditioned stimulus (for example a bell) with an unconditioned stimulus (for example food), as described above. In operant conditioning, however, the behaviour is not a part of the animal's repertoire of behaviour. The deliberate or otherwise use of reinforcement will result in a new behaviour.

In 1957, Skinner postulated a behavioural explanation for the acquisition of language in children. He argued that if an infant's vocalising was positively reinforced, then that infant would increase the frequency of that behaviour. Skinner (1957) outlined three ways in which the process of language acquisition might be achieved, as shown in Box 2.7.

Although greatly simplified the process outlined demonstrates how the behavioural model would

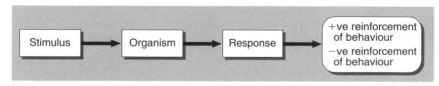

Fig 2.3 Operant conditioning

attempt to explain the acquisition of language in order to communicate.

The application of behaviourism

Operant conditioning, as an approach to understanding learning and behaviour, has had an enormous impact upon nursing and the ways in which some client groups are cared for. One behavioural treatment used in the field of mental health, for phobic conditions, is systematic desensitisation. This technique comprises pairing a response that inhibits anxiety, for example muscle relaxation, with something that provokes anxiety. Consider the case of an individual suffering from arachnophobia (a fear of spiders). In desensitisation a therapist would pair

the anxiety-provoking event in a graduated manner with relaxation techniques. So, for example, a therapist would commence desensitisation by showing the patient a photograph of a spider coupled with relaxation exercises. Eventually the therapist would show the patient a living spider and perhaps get him to touch the spider, again coupled with relaxation exercises. In between these two extremes are a series of graduated stimuli that could cause a corresponding graduated fear response and this is shown in Figure 2.4.

However, repeated pairing of the stimuli with relaxation would eventually bring about a different response to fear at the sight of spiders. Instead a patient would feel more comfortable and relaxed, because they would associate the relaxation with the spider instead of the anxiety and fear.

For a detailed description of this type of therapeutic intervention the reader is advised to see Paul and Bernstein (1976). Bellack et al (1982) have described the use of behaviourism as a mediator in a number of studies of social skills training for schizophrenic patients. They suggested that social skills were deficient in schizophrenic patients, resulting in social isolation. One study comprised targeting and improving the assertiveness of two chronic schizophrenic patients. Eye contact, speech duration, smiles, requests and compliances were reinforced positively. Results demonstrated that the targeted behaviours significantly improved and that these improvements remained for some weeks after the skills training.

Another example of the use of behavioural interventions to improve communication is recorded by Lovass (1976). A series of steps was taken to

---

Box 2.7 A behavioural explanation for language acquisition

1. Echoic response: here the infant mimics a noise made by others, who in turn reinforce the infant's behaviour.

2. Mand response: the infant engages in initiating sound but without meaning. The meaning is attached by others, once again reinforcement of the behaviour is provided by others.

3. Tact response: at this stage the child moves on to make an attempt to use a word to name something that is present in its environment. When the child successfully does this its behaviour is reinforced.

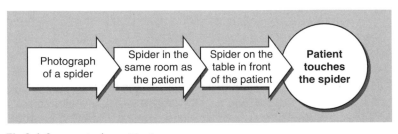

Fig 2.4 Systematic desensitisation

Table 2.1 Characteristics of the psychodynamic, behavioural and humanistic models

Issues	Psychodynamic (O-R) model	Behavioural model	Humanistic model
Philosophical view of the person	Basic drive is to relate to others and things. The person is the author and product of experience	All behaviour is learned in response to environmental reinforcement	Positive view of human beings. Drive towards becoming fully functioning
Internal v. external orientation	Dynamic interaction between inner and outer experience	Emphasis on external stimuli and measurable behaviour	Congruence between inner and outer experience is the ideal
Self concept	Various interpretations and emphases across several workers	Observable and measurable focus. Therefore self is largely ignored	Key, central concept. Self is involved in thought, feeling and behaviour
States of awareness	The unconscious is a central concept. Dynamic interplay between conscious and unconscious processes	Awareness and insight not central ideas	Accepts unconscious but focuses on the here and now
Feeling, thought and behaviour	Dynamic interplay between all three	Behaviour is central focus	Felt experience primary. Congruence between all three in the present is the ideal
Role of past, present and future	Past and present in constant dynamic interaction	Focus on the present and the future	Congruence can only be experienced in the present moment

train autistic children in vocal imitation. In Step 1, the therapist increased the child's vocalisations by reinforcing him (usually with food) contingent on such behaviour. In Step 2, the child was trained in temporal discrimination: his vocalisations were reinforced only if they were in response to the therapist's speech, i.e. if they occurred within five seconds of the therapist's vocalisation. In Step 3, finer discriminations were reinforced. For example, the child was reinforced for making successively closer approximations to the therapist's speech until he could match the particular sound given by the therapist. Lovass (1976) continued with a detailed account of how new behaviour was reinforced leading to increased vocalisation in the children.

Whereas the above examples draw from early experiments in this area they are given because the basic principles of behaviourism can be clearly identified. It is the case that these principles continue to be interpreted in contemporary behavioural work that still uses the stimulus response

relationship as central to any intervention. This can be illustrated by more contemporary literature (see, for example, McCue (2000) concerning behavioural interventions for people with learning disability in distressed states and Barr et al (2000) for an account of the use of structured teaching with children with autistic spectrum disorder). The examples given serve to demonstrate how a behaviourist view of the person may influence the ways in which nurses potentially communicate with their patients (Table 2.1).

Having briefly outlined the behavioural approach to understanding the person let us now consider the third of the three approaches outlined in this chapter, the humanistic model.

THE HUMANISTIC MODEL

Atkinson et al (1999) have suggested that during the first half of the 20th century the psychodynamic and behavioural approaches to understanding the person were dominant. However, during the late 1950s and early 1960s a group of psychologists developed a new and radical approach based on phenomenology in which the humanistic approach to understanding the person is central. Phenomenology rejects the behavioural approach to understanding the person where behaviour is seen as the result of associations or connections between stimuli and responses. It also rejects the suggestion that behaviour is controlled by unconscious impulses, located in our past, as suggested by the psychodynamic approach. Instead, humanism asserts the unique, subjective and lived experience of each individual.

From the humanistic approach came the work of Maslow (1954) who describes a system of hierarchy of needs in the person. These needs range from basic physiological needs such as food, water and air to complex psychological needs such as security, belonging and self-esteem. The pinnacle of this hierarchy is self-actualisation: the individual's need to find fulfillment and develop to his own potential.

Another important contributor to the humanistic approach is Carl Rogers. His ideas emerged from his therapeutic work with people in need of psychotherapy. He believed that people have an innate tendency to develop and grow in maturity, which will lead an individual to actualise all the capacities she has. If a person's development is stunted it is likely that it is due to relationships in which their experiencing was denied, defined or discounted. What is healing is a relationship in which a person feels fully accepted and valued, the famous core conditions for therapeutic change viz. unconditional positive regard (acceptance), empathy and genuineness. Central to this approach is a fundamental philosophical belief in the individual to develop to his full potential. Atkinson et al (1999) has offered the four principles outlined in Box 2.8, which characterise the humanistic outlook of the person.

Two excellent examples of how the humanistic approach affects the ways in which nurses and

---

Box 2.8 The four principles of humanism

1. *The person is of central interest.*
   Humanists assert that people are not merely objects that respond to their environment when suitably reinforced. Rather people are dynamic interactive beings who are able to shape their environment as well as respond to it.

2. *Aspects of human behaviour are important to investigation.*
   Central to humanism is the idea of the quest for fulfilment and self actualisation as described by Rogers (1970). Human choice and creativity are important parts of this.

3. *Subjectivity is more important than objectivity.*
   Understanding the lived experience of people is essential. Humanists argue that the rigours of other schools of psychology distort the nature of human experience in the pursuit of objectivity.

4. *The value of the person.*
   Great value is placed upon the integrity and uniqueness of the individual. Humanists believe that the objective of psychology should be to understand the individual and should not be concerned with controlling and manipulating the person.

---

other therapists communicate with people can be found in the specialism of learning disabilities. It will be seen from the examples given that the principles of humanism have the potential to affect the type of relationship between health care professionals and the person being cared for.

Behavioural difficulties and learning disabilities

For many years the most dominant form of therapeutic intervention for behavioural difficulties was based upon behaviourism. That is, therapeutic programmes were developed for individuals that

Box 2.9 Gentle Teaching: four core themes

1. *Unconditional valuing.*
   Gentle teaching asserts the importance of valuing the person and the giving of non contingent reinforcement as opposed to behaviourism, where reinforcement is contingent upon desired behaviour.

2. *Teaching the client to value others.*
   The person is taught to return this unconditional valuing to others, not purely as a response to reinforcement but as part of the interdependence of people.

3. *Changing the attitudes of carers.*
   Menolascino and McGee recognised the need to change the attitudes of staff caring for people with challenging behaviour to become more enlightened and develop closer bonds between them and the people being cared for.

4. *Human engagement.*
   Lastly McGee points to the need for meaningful interaction between people that fully engages them, i.e. that human beings need to relate to one another as human beings in committed relationships.

individuals. Unlike behavioural approaches the provision of 'rewards' does not depend upon a demonstration of desirable behaviours sought by the therapist. Gentle Teaching would appear to comprise four core themes outlined in Box 2.9. It is fair to say that there is considerable debate about the legitimacy and efficacy of such interventions (Jones & Connell 1993). Notwithstanding the criticisms that have been made, Gentle Teaching is an excellent example of how a particular view or theory of a person impacts upon the ways in which nurses and therapists communicate and interact with people with learning disabilities.

 Activity 2.1 An exercise in Gentle Teaching

The reader is invited to spend some time reflecting upon Gentle Teaching and then identify those characteristics that suggest its practice and ideology to be grounded in the humanistic perspective of the person.

reinforced desirable behaviours and punished or ignored undesirable behaviours. In the early 1980s two researchers (Menolascino & McGee 1991) from the University of Nebraska challenged this approach as inappropriate. They argued that the behavioural approach did not respect the integrity and uniqueness of people with a learning disability who were a devalued group. They promoted instead an enlightened approach known as Gentle Teaching.

Gentle Teaching

This form of therapeutic intervention comprises a range of strategies that uses nonaversive techniques. The principal aim is to develop bonding between

Normalisation (social role valorisation)
Wolfensberger (1972) has stated that 'people with a mental handicap have the same rights and, wherever possible, the same responsibilities as other people of the same age in any given society'. This valuing and enlightened outlook of the individual was clearly in keeping with the humanist perspective of the person. Nowhere were the underlying ideological principles of normalisation more clearly articulated than by Grunewald (1969) who said:

The principle of normalisation is applicable both to the development of the retarded individual [adult or child] and to the needs of parents – the validity of this principle is not negated by the fact that the majority of mentally handicapped persons cannot become fully adjusted to society. The term implies rather a striving in various ways towards what is normal. Even the most severely handicapped person can thus be normalised in one or more respects. Normalisation does not imply any denial of the person's handicap. It involves rather exploiting his other mental and physical capabilities so that his handicap becomes less pronounced. It also means that he has the same rights and obligations as other people, as near as possible. (Grunewald 1969)

Seven core themes of normalisation can be identified and these are detailed in Box 2.10 and briefly described below.

The role of consciousness and unconsciousness in service provision. Much of the work of health care professionals can be conducted on an unconscious level, without sensitivity towards the ways in which their own values affect the nature of interaction and communication with the people they care for. These unconscious values may originate from early experience, as described earlier in the psychodynamic approach. Normalisation challenges carers to become acutely conscious of how their values, language and beliefs about people with a learning disability may adversely affect their care. Such a theme is extremely important to the health of people with learning disabilities it has long been

---

Box 2.10 The core themes of normalisation

1. The role of consciousness and unconsciousness in services.
2. The relevance of role expectancy and role circularity.
3. The conservatism corollary.
4. The developmental model.
5. The power of imitation.
6. The dynamics and relevance of social imagery.
7. The importance of social integration and participation.

---

known that people with learning disabilities have poorer health than that of the general population and often experience prejudice from health care professionals (Gates 1998).

The relevance of role expectancy and role circularity. It is often the case that people have low expectations of those with learning disabilities. This may serve to reinforce a person's disability because low expectation, in this context, results in reduced learning that in itself reinforces the nature of learning disability. When interacting with people with learning disabilities this is something that health care professionals should bear in mind. Normalisation has sought to promote positive role expectations by reinforcing the role of people with learning disabilities that will break the vicious circle of low expectation and therefore low performance.

The conservatism corollary. This can best be described as when a person has a characteristic that is not generally valued in society and that when this occurs everything possible should be done to minimise that characteristic. A concrete example of this core theme might be a carer encouraging a person with learning disabilities, who persistently dribbles, to use a range of strategies to reduce the amount of dribbling for example, by attention to posture, breathing exercises and the use of tissues.

The developmental model. This core theme promotes the potential for growth and development in all individuals. It is clearly in keeping with the humanistic belief in self-actualisation. To achieve such a core theme it would be important to ensure that all service-providing agencies made for adequate provision to meet the lifelong learning needs of people with learning disabilities.

The power of imitation. This theme acknowledges the importance of imitation or modelling to learning. Clearly during normal development much learning is achieved through imitating the behaviour of other significant people, for example brothers, sisters and friends. For the person with learning disabilities there is no exception and it is imperative that good role models are available in a person's life so that they have adequate opportunities for learning.

The dynamics and relevance of social imagery. Learning disability has shouldered a negative imagery for many years. This theme acknowledges that this state of affairs must be tackled by identifying negative imagery and replacing it with more positive imagery. There has been much work undertaken in this area by the Royal Society for Mentally Handicapped People (Mencap).

The importance of social integration and participation. In the past it was the case that people with learning disabilities were segregated from others because of institutional care. The recent White Paper – *Valuing People* (DoH 2001) outlines central government policy for people with learning disabilities. This is based upon the four principles of rights, independence, choice and inclusion. The issue of inclusion is an important factor for all health professionals because it is envisaged that people with learning disabilities will access all mainstream services. Never before has the issue of communication and interpersonal skill been so important for working with this client group. Since the 1970s there have been developments in the practical implementation of normalisation and, in service provision the concept of normalisation has greatly affected the ways in which people with a learning disability are cared for. The principles of normalisation, when applied to service provision are both interesting and important. Since the inception of normalisation in the late 1950s normalisation principles as a distinct entity have, to a greater or lesser extent, been applied in the UK since the 1970s and the core value – that people with learning disabilities have the same human value as everyone else – can now be found in virtually every service statement regarding planning and the delivery of services in the UK. However, to achieve the ideal of the same rights and, wherever possible, the same responsibilities as others continues to be extremely problematic.

Activity 2.2 An exercise to explore the concept of normalisation

Identify three reasons why the ideals of normalisation might be difficult to achieve for a man with profound learning disability. You may wish to make reference to the recent White Paper – *Valuing People* (DoH 2001).

Although these core themes have been applied to learning disabilities, it is not inappropriate to apply them to other groups of people who may be devalued, for example, the older person or those with mental health problems. This powerful concept has the potential to challenge health care professionals to explore how they communicate with people and to seek alternative more enlightened ways of working with those who are devalued.

CONCLUSION

This chapter has put human beings centrestage in the study of the nature of communication, that is what and how do people communicate? We have seen that different models of the person rest on different underlying assumptions. Readers will, we hope, now be in a better position to reflect on their own assumptions about people when communicating with them and will be conscious of the choices available from sources other than their own experiences. It is a basic theme of this book that with understanding and awareness it is possible to be more intentional, and hence more effective, in one's communication with others. We now turn to the wider social context in which human contact takes place to investigate its influence on communication.

REFERENCES

Atkinson RL, Atkinson RC, Smith EE, Bem DJ, Hilgard ER 1999 Introduction to psychology, 13th edn. Harcourt Brace Jovanovich, London

Balint M 1964 The doctor, his patient and the illness, 2nd edn. Tavistock/Routledge, London

Barr O et al 2000 Structured teaching. In: Gates B, Gear J, Wray J (eds) Behavioural distress: concepts and strategies. Baillière Tindall, Edinburgh

Bellack A, Hersen M, Kazdin A 1982 International handbook of behaviour modification and therapy. Plenum Press, New York

DoH 2001 Valuing people: A new strategy for learning disability for the 21st century. Cm 5086. HMSO, London

Gates B 1998 A new health agenda for learning disabled people: Reflections on platitudes and political rhetoric. Journal of Learning Disabilities for Nursing, Health and Social Care 2(1): 1–2

Grunewald K 1969 The mentally retarded in Sweden. In: Recent advances in the study of subnormality, 2nd edn. National Association for Mental Retardation, London

Jones R, Connell E 1993 Ten years of gentle teaching: much ado about nothing? The Psychologist Dec: 544–548

Klein M 1963 Our adult world and its roots in infancy. Pitman, London

Maslow A 1954 Motivation and personality. Harper and Row, New York

McCue M 2000 Behavioural interventions. In Gates B, Gear J, Wray J (eds) Behavioural distress: concepts and strategies. Baillière Tindall, Edinburgh

Menolascino FJ, McGee JJ 1991 Beyond gentle teaching: a non-aversive approach to helping those in need. Plenum Press, New York

Noonan E 1983 Counseling young people. Methuen, London

Paul G, Bernstein D 1976 Anxiety and clinical problems: systematic desensitisation and related techniques. In: Spence J, Carson R, Thibaut (eds) 1976 Behavioural approaches to therapy. General Learning Press, New Jersey

Pavlov I 1902 The work of the digestive glands. Translated by WH Thompson. Charles Griffin, London

Pervin LA 1993 Personality: theory and research, 6th edn. John Wiley, New York

Rogers CR 1970 On becoming a person: a therapist's view of psychotherapy. Houghton Mifflin, Boston

Rogers CR 1974 On becoming a person, 4th edn. Constable, London

Skinner BF 1938 The behaviour of organisms. Appleton-Century Crofts, New York

Watson JB 1924 Behaviourism (revised edition, 1930). In: Stevenson L (ed) 1974 Seven theories of human nature. Oxford University Press, Oxford

Wolfensberger W 1972 Normalisation. National Institute of Mental Retardation, Toronto

FURTHER READING

Freud A 1986 The ego and the mechanisms of defence. Hogarth Press, London

Medcof J, Roth L (eds) 1979 Approaches to psychology. Oxford University Press, Milton Keynes

Ruddock R (ed) 1972 Six approaches to the person. Routledge, London

Stevenson L 1981 The study of human nature. Oxford University Press, Oxford

Winnicott DW 1988 Human nature. Free Association Books, London

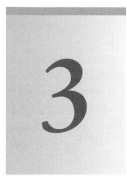

Social factors affecting communication

Peter Morrall

INTRODUCTION

Someone comes up to you in a bar or cafe and says to you 'Hello, how are you?'. What does this person mean by this phrase? Is it simply a 'neutral' and concise greeting that can be taken at 'face-value' on the basis of the explicit meaning intended by that individual, which unambiguously corresponds with the meaning accepted by you? Even if the nonverbal messages coinciding with the question (a smile, gesture of the hand, slight movement of the legs, and tone of voice) have to be taken into consideration, is that all there is to understanding this communication?

To demonstrate the ways in which social factors affect the meaning of what is said and how it is received, reflect on the differences in the communication event if the 'Hello, how are you?' is said to you by a man or woman, or someone from a different ethnic group, religious group, and/or, age group, a police officer in uniform, the collector of your household refuge, your general practitioner, or your employer. What if the venue is a 'singles' meeting place; a 'family'-oriented setting, or a gay/lesbian scene? What if it is in a village, or the busy inner city? What if the 'hello' is voiced by someone dressed in a similar fashion to a notorious terrorist who recently had been portrayed as extremely dangerous in the news? How might your reaction be affected if currently there is a media panic about 'a mad axemen' at large in the area?

Furthermore, is the 'question' element 'how are you?' really a query about your state of health, or a socially acceptable greeting, which invites an equally socially acceptable response such as 'Okay thank you, how are you?' Try to test this the next time

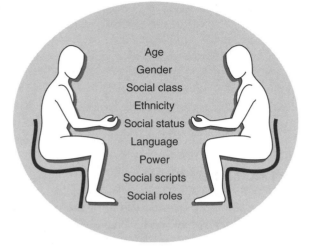

Fig 3.1 Social factors influencing interpersonal communication

you are propositioned with 'Hello, how are you?' by explaining in great and laborious detail your bio-psycho-social-spiritual health strengths and deficits. My guess is that you will not be communicated with so readily by this person in the future! However, in other cultures (for example, there may be differences between North America and Europe) or in other situations (such as when in discussion with a medical practitioner or a close family member) this greeting/question would indeed elicit a more expansive retort and this would be highly appropriate. It is the social context that (in part) dictates what significance the greeting/question has for the individuals involved.

Hence, communicating with other humans is considerably more complicated than it may at first seem. There are the obvious problems in understanding the explicit words and nonverbal behaviour, as well as the implicit messages that are being used by the people involved. However, apart from these interpersonal factors, communication is linked to the social environment in which it is taking place, and is affected by the social identity of those who are participating (Hartley 1993, McQuail 1984) (Fig. 3.1).

To fully comprehend communicative interchanges between humans, the social context in

communication has to be appreciated and its implications taken into account. Moreover, although not the focus of this chapter, the effects of evolutionary and biological predispositions on human behaviour, along with social factors, are also involved in forming the psychological (intrapersonal) conditions of communication.

When a student nurse commences a new clinical experience, and introduces herself to a patient whom she has never met before, both are sending and receiving important signals about each other's social identity. Signals of identity, such as respective ages, gender, ethnic grouping, and status in society may influence the type of communication that takes place. Each identifies the other in a particular role, the student identifying the other person in the role of 'patient', and the patient perceiving the student in the role of 'nurse'.

Communication between professional colleagues will involve the same process of recognising each other's social attributes. Although age and gender still affect the form that the communication will take, what predominates at work is the prestige, power, and control that each nurse is ascribed by the organisation (and ultimately by society).

Whatever and however people communicate it is not done in a neutral way. Messages sent verbally or nonverbally are moderated to comply with the norms of the society to which we belong. The communication that occurs at an interpersonal level is not conducted in a social vacuum. Nurses need to reflect upon the immediate and wider social context in which a communication takes place to fully understand what it implies.

FREEDOM?

One of the key sociological questions concerning interpersonal communication is 'Are we free to communicate, or is the form and content of our communication predetermined by society'?

As Hartley has observed, there is 'something of a battle between those who regard society as the backdrop against which humans choose to act and

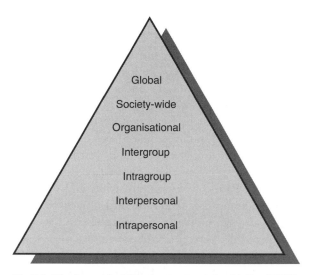

Fig 3.2 The Pyramid of Communication (after McQuail 2000)

those who feel that society creates or determines the ways in which we act' (1993, p. 80).

McQuail (2000) suggested that society organises different levels of communication. These levels, for McQuail, can be considered in a hierarchy, which he represents as a pyramid (Fig. 3.2). At the pinnacle of the pyramid, McQuail proposed, is 'society-wide' communication. Here mass media systems such as television, film, and video/DVD, transmit messages about cultural norms and deviancy as entertainment or education.

However, I have added a higher level to illustrate the importance of global communication, particularly with respect to electronic systems, that is the Internet, mobile and landline telephones, and faxes. Moreover, countries have trading, monetary, cultural, and political ties with groups of other countries and have supranational bureaucracies (such as the European Union) transmitting policy directives and laws. Large numbers of people travel abroad for holidays, move across continents as refugees, migrant workers, and as students studying at foreign universities or taking a 'gap year'. There are also international nongovernmental organisations, such as the World Health Organisation, Medicines Sans Frontiers, the Red Cross and the World Bank, that dispatch advice about, for example, health

and finances. Therefore, communication leaks from and through, national boundaries.

Below these two levels there are the networks of communication associated with social institutions (for example, schools and universities; health promotion agencies; political parties and governments, and large-scale business organisations. These social institutions communicate details of their activities both externally (for example, reporting to outside monitors of quality, funding agencies, and the government; advertising their products to target client/customer groups) and internally (for example, in-house policies discussed and delivered verbally, in writing and electronically).

Next is the intergroup level at which community-based groups operate. That is, there is formal and informal communication between, for example, local administrative agencies, associations, and commercial outlets. This is followed by the level of communication that occurs within the elemental human groupings of a society (essentially the family and peer assemblages).

All of the levels mentioned so far to a greater or lesser extent 'shape' (and to some degree therefore control) interpersonal communication. Below these 'social' levels, are the 'personal' levels. The interpersonal level includes all intimate relationships. For McQuail, intrapersonal communication refers to the individual's psychological and physiological mechanisms that process information both in terms of receiving messages and delivering messages.

We may believe that at these personal levels we are freely, consciously, and meaningfully making decisions about what to transmit to others, and what sense to make of what is transmitted to us. But, the process of 'shaping' emerging from the preceding communication levels will set the scene for what can and what can't be communicated by the individual. Furthermore, communication flows between levels within the pyramidal structure (for example, government with business; individual consumers with retail stores in their area). But it also jumps levels (for example, mass communication is designed to reach the population as a whole but ultimately it is the individual who clues-in to what is being 'sold' (whether the product is goods or information). Moreover, there is also considerable overlap between the intragroup and interpersonal levels. For example, family members communicate with other members as individuals perhaps about issues that are not directly related to the family. Crucially, what is being thought by the individual prior and during communication from the social deterministic viewpoint is constructed by concepts handed-down by his/her culture. We cannot discuss with another person ideas that do not make reference to the material and abstract concepts, which already have existence, or at least have a pre-existing conceptual backdrop from which apparently new thoughts have emerged 'from nowhere'.

Social considerations will dictate the content, style and outcome of the communication that occurs between individuals. The conversational interaction between a nurse and a service user or a professional colleague are preorganised by each participant's gender, identity, age, ethnic origin, educational background and overall status in society.

An 18-year-old female student nurse and a 60-year-old male senior partner of a large legal firm who is in hospital with a myocardial infarction, will find it hard to ignore the social attributes, experience, and culturally constructed view on life (and death) that each has, and to have a socially uncontaminated interchange of opinions. They seemingly talk 'freely' to each other but their thinking, words, bodily movements, and interpretative skills are limited by the difference in their social status (principally, their age, gender and occupation).

However, the eminent sociologist Anthony Giddens (1984) has attempted to show that whilst human behaviour is not totally under the control of the individual, nor is it completely modelled by society. Giddens tried to bridge the gap between those theorists who believe that people act voluntarily, that is they have free choice over what they do, and those theorists who argue that human behaviour is completely determined by society. It is the synthesis of the two extremes of voluntarism and determinism, as advocated by Giddens, which may be the most appropriate theoretical

approach to understanding interpersonal communication. That is, humans do have choice in what they think, do and say, but this is constrained in varying degrees by social factors. The nurse's interaction with service users and colleagues will be controlled in part by the personal attributes of all of those concerned, for example their attitudes, personality and intellect, as well as by such socially prescribed attributes as 'role' and 'status'. Individuals, therefore, belong to a society that has a pregiven structure. Rules, written laws, roles and relationships make up this structure, and unwritten regulations determine what is acceptable, and what is unacceptable, behaviour. The structure exists only in the abstract sense, but provides a framework that supports and governs all human activities.

The proposition that the framework of society operates robustly over individual volition is contested by those holding the view that our biological make-up is the potent determinant. Lewis Wolpert (2002) professor of biology as applied to medicine of University College London, has reasoned that the social environment acts on behaviour that is already genetically compelled. For Wolpert, the fact that human language is universal is indicative of our biological heritage. Neurological circuits, developed in embryo, enable us to talk, although the content of speech will be inspired by the culture in which we live. Significantly however, biological scientists belonging to the 'genome project' (that is the mapping of the genetic make-up of the human body) have accepted the major influence society has on how we behave. That is, humans are far more prisoners of the social environment than their biological inheritance (McKie 2001).

This is not to assume that social determinism is inevitable and a replacement for biological dominion over human actions and thoughts. Arguably, there is a reflexive relationship between the social agent and the social system. What individuals communicate is inspired by, but also inspiring to, the society to which they belong (Giddens 1991). We both verbalise and signify societal norms and assist in the creation of these norms through our communication.

Activity 3.1 Communication levels

Draw the amended version of McQuail's (2000) communication pyramid.

Enter within each level examples of communication that involve you personally. Indicate on the drawing how your examples are interconnected.

POWER

Power is the ability of individuals or groups to make their own interests or concerns count, even when others resist... Power is an element of almost all social relationships.... (*Giddens 2001, p. 420*)

Power inevitably enters into the interpersonal communication nexus. That is, a lack of social power may be associated with a lack of power when communicating with others.

Power is a pivotal element to the structure of a society and in human interchanges. People, categorised by such social traits as economic class, gender, ethnicity, wealth and occupation, have differing degrees of influence in society generally, but also perhaps over their own lives. More and more the 'society' in question here is not the nation state (for example, the United Kingdom, Zimbabwe or Australia), but 'superstates' (for example, the European Union), and ultimately a globalised economy and culture (Miles 2001).

An individual who is unemployed and impoverished in Sudan has little social power, whereas the Chairperson of a multibillion dollar transnational media, biochemical, or armaments corporation, has a considerable amount of capacity to influence. A male hospital manager in the United Kingdom conversing with a female staff nurse on a medical ward may have more power allocated to him because of gender identity and work-related role. Therefore, he is more likely to achieve his goal

of reducing costs than the staff nurse who seeks an increase in resources.

Although these structural elements in society (for example, employment status, wealth–poverty circumstances) regulate human behaviour to a significant degree, as Giddens (1991) has suggested, individual human action influences the structure of society. The individual in Sudan and the United Kingdom staff nurse have some potential influence. The former could engage in a political campaign for international aid or revolution. The latter could, given her specific knowledge about the quality of care in her clinical area, negotiate with the manager, and recruit other puissant colleagues to support her viewpoint.

French and Raven (1959), and Collins and Raven (1969) have chronicled a number of different sources of socially manufactured power. I have provided examples within their typology of how social power is involved in interpersonal communication:

1. Expert power: where it is assumed that someone has greater knowledge and skills than ourselves because of long training or experience. Those with expert power communicate their authority nonverbally (for example, the wearing of a uniform by nurses and white coats by hospital-based doctors; the archetypal horn-rim glasses and large desk of the general practitioner; 'academic-dress' worn by university teachers), and verbally (for example, the accumulation and transmission of esoteric knowledge by medical and nursing consultants and teachers).

2. Coercive power: where control is exercised physically over others. Parents, police officers, prison officers and mental health nurses may indicate verbally that they are about to prevent the movements of their 'target' by giving a verbal warning. Their nonverbal behaviour when, for example, restraining a disruptive individual, is usually unambiguously indicative of the desire to compel that person to stop his/her disruptive actions. Literally, that person is prevented from moving.

3. Reward power: where emotional or tangible payments are given in order to modify or stop

what others are doing or saying (for example, nurses caring for people with learning disabilities may use words of praise and approval, and/or signs such as a smile or touch, to reward and therefore encourage the learning of a new skill).

4. Legitimate power: where another person (for example, a judge, police officer, medical practitioner) has the authority to influence others, and this authority has been permitted by a legitimate source such as a government. In a similar way to expertise, legitimacy may be communicated by uniform (as with a 'beat' police officer, traffic/community warden, and soldier), or a badge-of-office (for example, the warrant card of the plain-clothed police officer; the name/title plate of the school headteacher and university professor; the ward-sister's label pinned to her chest). Alternatively, legitimate power may be inferred through speech (for example, the prime minister's, president's or monarch's address to the nation; the consultant surgeon's oration about a patient's condition during the ward round).

5. Referent power: where another person has the skills, attitudes, or intelligence that we wish we had ourselves, and we testify to the superiority of that person through our attitudes. This may be communicated through overt expressions of deference and reverence to the point of sycophancy (for example, 'I wish I was like him/her'; 'She knows how to deal with problems, we should ask her'). On the other hand, more subtle messages of reference, implying awe, may be conveyed (for example, in multidisciplinary meetings involving health care personnel, nursing and paramedical staff may await the medical consultant's opinion before, heavily swayed by that opinion, deciding on particular approaches to care).

6. Informational power: where, in the 'information age', easy and sweeping access to knowledge (especially via the Internet) becomes indispensable in gaining high educational qualifications, good employment conditions, financial security, and consumer satisfaction. Informational power is demonstrated in our ability to use data to win arguments (for example, when nurses, doctors, and other clinicians are debating over the appropriate care for a health service user; the health service user visiting his/her general practitioner armed with the results from all of the recent clinical trials on a certain treatment he/she is demanding to be prescribed).

Power in interpersonal relations exists, therefore, when an individual behaves in such a way that it will produce a change in another individual or individuals (Dowding 1996), and this ability will depend on the social status of all concerned. A hospital nurse (in his/her relatively socially prestigious role), by explaining the ward routine, details of treatment to a patient (in his/her relatively low-status role) has the power to reduce the patient's anxiety about being in hospital. The community nurse who demonstrates to the patient how to self-medicate has the power to reduce the patient's reliance on professional assistance.

McQuail (1984) has indicated a number of generalisations that may be made about the ways in which power can be exploited through communication. Monopolising the conversation can have the effect of gaining control and achieving a desired outcome. Where dominance occurs, and goes unchallenged, the greater the influence. A person can ensure a message is accepted by making it coincide with the beliefs of the other person. The content of the message will also be important in determining how influential the communicator will be. For example, the influence will be greater if the topic under discussion is about an issue with which the other person has no personal experience. Someone who is regarded as credible and having high status, through being physically attractive, intellectually admired and with much in common with the audience, will be far more powerful than someone who has less visible and psychological attributes.

Being a patient and a student nurse carries a relatively low amount of prestige in health care organisations compared to that received by the qualified health care professionals. Both the patient and the student nurse are in a different structural position (in terms of their status in the organisational hierarchy) to that of the qualified staff.

Moreover, the qualified members of staff are seen as permanent, whereas the patient and the student are viewed as transient. If the patient or student nurse is also disliked because of an unpleasant personality, and is perceived to be endowed with restricted physical beauty, then it is very unlikely that person will be listened to with the same degree of application as, for example, the resident modern matron who has an engaging personality and comely physique!

However, the social prescription of power is mutable. Society confers power but can renounce power. That is, power can be removed from those who have it. In the health arena, patients are now becoming more assertive in their dealings with medical personnel.

Powerfulness is accrued to a much greater extent when others acquiesce, and this is demonstrated well in the traditional 'sick role'. For a medical practitioner to be so dominant in the doctor–patient relationship the patient must adopt a passive form of interaction.

Activity 3.2 The use and exploitation of power in communication

Observe the ways in which you, other nurses, and doctors exercise power by controlling the content and style of what is communicated when in discussion with service users. What influence do the physical characteristics of the participants have on these occasions?

SICKNESS

Talcott Parsons (1951) argued that there is a type of socially acceptable behaviour for people who are ill. Parsons suggests that illness itself is a form of deviant behaviour, which has to be regulated in order that society can continue to operate effectively. Too much uncontrolled illness in society would lead to major social disruption. There would not

be enough people to work or carry out family responsibilities.

The sick role, for Parsons, is regarded as a 'contract' between the person who is ill and the rest of society, the latter being represented by the health care professionals. Control over access to the sick role is conducted in particular by medical practitioners, although increasingly nurses working in the surgeries of general practitioners are delegated some elements of this process, and therefore they are also involved in deciding who is and who isn't legitimately sick. Indeed the British Medical Association has advocated that nurses take over much of the 'gate-keeping' function for the sick role due to the mounting bureaucratic demands on general practitioners, the large number of trivial ailments brought by patients, and the falling numbers of doctors working in this area of work (Laurance 2002).

When an individual enters the sick role he/she is given a number of privileges by society, but also has a number of obligations to society. The sick person is exempt from work and family responsibilities, and is not blamed for being ill. However, he/she must seek and follow medical advice, and must want to recover as quickly as possible.

There is much debate about how realistic Parson's concept of the sick role is in today's society (Morrall 2001). With reference to interpersonal communication, the concept does point to a social pressure on patients to perform in a special communicative mode once they have accepted the role of being sick. If patients want to be regarded as having a legitimate illness they are encouraged to accept the treatment offered by those involved in their care. As a consequence of an individual entering into the sick role, with its concomitant obligations and rights, verbal and nonverbal behaviour would tend to be inert thereby indicating compliance.

Parson's model of the sick role was adjusted by Szasz and Hollender (1956). Szasz and Hollender portrayed the doctor–patient relationship as much more potentially dynamic for the patient than had been projected by Parsons (see Table 3.1). They accepted that in certain 'sick role' states, when the patient is not full cognisant (for example, during major surgery, if extremely toxaemic, deeply depressed, psychotic, severely senile, or suffering physiological shock) her/his interactive responses will be stifled or incoherent. Here the power of the practitioner is absolute. But, for many if not most illnesses, and for much of the duration of contact, patients can engage in discussions about their treatment with medical directions either on the basis of 'participation' or 'co-operation'.

However, in a tacit admission of the medical practitioners continued unreliability to help create the condition through which patient-activity is possible (many decades after Szasz and Hollender indicted that this was both possible and desirable), Sir Peter Morris, President of the Royal College of Surgeons in the UK, accepted that surgeons working in the NHS were failing to communicate effectively with their patients:

> *Communication requires time, awareness and skills from the surgeon, and good patient information [that's] comprehensible ... in reality, such time is not available, because of the pressure to see more patients and the lack of manpower. (Morris reported in Boseley 2001)*

Morris's comments were made following the formal report into medical practice at Bristol Royal Infirmary where adequate information was not provided to parents about the risks of what was to be found to be 'inappropriate' heart surgery on their babies.

The degree to which a patient is active whilst communicating with health care professionals will be consequent on the social grouping of the sufferer. That is patient empowerment may be more common amongst middle-class, articulate, professional groups than those without substantial educational and social capital to draw upon.

Moreover, a patient's communicative involvement in his/her treatment may be encouraged or discouraged depending upon the cultural affiliation between doctor and patient (Freidson 1970). A white, female, middle-aged medical practitioner is more likely to share equally communicative interchanges with a white, middle-aged lawyer than a black, unemployed youth.

> **Activity 3.3** Forms of interpersonal communication
>
> Use Szasz and Hollender's model (Table 3.1) to evaluate your own communication interactions with a selection of health service users. Reflect on what forms of communication are taking place, and what forms you believe should occur.

DISCOURSE

Socially constructed bias, therefore, is pervasive in interpersonal communication. The intent of those who have power in society and in relationships is often achieved through manipulating or 'distorting' communication (Malhotra 1987). Patterns of communication emerge as a consequence of the languages and technologies developed by powerful factions in society for the purpose of 'mystifying'

Table 3.1 Interpersonal communication in sick roles (after Szasz & Hollender 1956)

Type of role adopted	Examples of communication
Active–passive (doctor is active, patient is passive)	No or little interpersonal communication between doctor and patient
Guidance–co-operation (doctor guides, patient co-operates)	The doctor communicates details of the diagnosis, treatment, and prognosis, and the patient indicates that he/she understands and complies
Mutual participation (doctor and patient negotiate openly)	The doctor offers alternative approaches to treatment, and the patient makes a choice

underlying status, jurisdiction, and ideological struggles. These factions include governments, political parties, religions, academic disciplines, as well as health disciplines such as medicine, nursing, clinical psychology, counselling, physiotherapy, pharmacology, and occupational therapy.

According to Jurgen Habermas (1970, 1972) what is communicated has the appearance of being understood, equitable and acceptable to each individual, but below the surface there may be a 'hidden agenda' which is directed by the person (or group) with power. Forms of communication, such as language, are organised to ensure an outcome that is in the interest of the powerful individual. It is denotative of the power of this individual that the communication process can be organised in this way.

Power-distorted communication is commonplace in the health care arena (Hugman 1991). For example, in the health service users are 'asked' to follow treatment regimes and alter their lifestyle habits. However, the agenda is not wholly or even partially that of the service user's but has been evoked by the goals and restrictions of professional and organisational practice, as well as economics and politics.

People with power have the ability to select the content and form of what is being communicated. This is done through particular symbols, practices, and styles of language that ensure domination. The organising of communication on the basis of power is described as 'discourse', and the variety of discourses those health care professionals embrace has been studied by Michel Foucault (1971, 1973, 1974, 1980). In particular Foucault examined how medical knowledge has been constructed to produce an apparently legitimate, and consequently prominent, way of viewing the world.

But Foucault's argument is that there is not one 'factual' way of viewing the world. Different societies, both historically and cross-culturally, have different realities. This line of reasoning would imply that seemingly real entities such as 'health' and 'disease' are not real at all. Diabetes, obesity, anorexia nervosa, hyperactivity, heart disease and dementia are arbitrary categories whose existence, boundaries and importance to both individuals and society have changed in the past and will change in the future. The way in which service users think and talk about their bodies is controlled by the concepts, theories and symbols that have been supplied by health care professionals. The medical discourse in turn is a reflection of what those with power in society have deemed to be of significance at that point in time.

Asking patients about their exercise, smoking and drinking habits, and encouraging them to take more responsibility for their health is not simply an example of good medical and nursing practice. These things are being discussed because of social, economic and political contingencies that lie beyond the face-to-face encounter between service user and health care professional. They are the consequence of such historical processes as the Enlightenment and industrialisation. Processes such as these gradually changed our attitudes about what was important in society from religion and 'the community' to a belief in the uniqueness and sanctity of the individual human being and the body (Brooks 1993).

Doctors use language, that is 'medical jargon', imagery, for example, the white coat, and technologies, for example, stethoscopes, sphygmomanometers, body scans, laboratory testing, psychological assessments, and genetic screening, in the application of their power on patients (Morrall 2001). Moreover, according to David Armstrong (1984), himself a medical practitioner and a sociologist, eliciting 'the patient's view' becomes a technique designed to furnish the doctor's influence over the patient rather than helping to empower the patient in her/his dealings with the doctor.

Armstrong points out that patients have since the late 18th century been asked to provide details of their conditions in order to nurture what Foucault (1973) described as the 'medical gaze'. However, the patient traditionally is asked to speak, and is listened to, but not heard beyond helping to confirm or repudiate the significance given to physical indications of disorder. Communicating with the patient is a form of interrogation through which the medical perspective, not the patient's, can be instituted. From this perspective, the 'patient's view' has been incorporated within the medical discourse.

Paradoxically, the service user's perspective has been adopted explicitly by other health care workers as a professional objective. The doctrine of 'patient empowerment' is now proliferated especially by nurses. The patient no longer can reside in the sanctity of the passive sick role but is encouraged (if not forced) to make treatment choices and take care of him/herself.

The most important element of discourse is language. The discipline of sociolinguistics explores how social factors moderate language. Language, as with all other forms of communication, is not context-free. There is a direct link between the manner of speech, the words used, and how society is structured (given that the propensity for humans to speak is biologically granted).

Membership of social groupings provides people with a particular form of linguistic expression. The way a person speaks may afford the listener an immediate clue as to the speaker's status in society and his/her social affiliations. Members of the British Royal family have verbal mannerisms that differ from the majority of the British population. In societies where there are multiple ethnic, tribal, or clan groupings, the way in which a common language (for example, English or Spanish) is accentuated and assembled can indicate the social identity of the speaker where skin colour and other corporeal properties are not sufficient.

Nurses are socialised to use a form of language that identifies them with other nurses and other health care professionals. They belong to a 'speech community' of nurses within which there is a sharing of verbal signs and professional jargon (Gumperz 1968). The use of the specialised language associated with health care will symbolise to colleagues group membership, and to others that they are excluded from that grouping (Miller & Form 1962). One form of speech, such as technical jargon, may predominate when nurses are amongst other nurses. Professionals speak differently, however, when they are involved with other speech communities. When nurses or doctors are with their families they will (or perhaps should) use words, phrases and intonations that are appropriate to the shared meanings that have developed in that social group rather than those they have learned in their professional role.

The very nature of the health system in Britain means that nurses communicate with service users and colleagues from diverse social class backgrounds. Members of different social classes have alternative ways of expressing themselves linguistically.

Social class divisions could be dissipating (Crook et al 1992), but their influence on verbal expression has traditionally been highly noticeable and may still be apparent. Research by Schatzman and Strauss (1955) in America indicated that there were significant variations between working- and middle-class use of language. The people who were designated as working class in the study talked of experiences with which they were familiar but the listener was not. They would not, however, attempt to 'clue in' the listener by giving background information. On the other hand, the middle-class participants did help the listener to understand by supplying extra details.

In Britain, research by Bernstein (1975) has implied a strong link between the social class to which an individual belongs and the form of speech in use. Bernstein argued that working-class people use a different linguistic code to that used by middle-class people. The former uses a restricted, or context-tied code whereas the latter make use of an elaborated code.

The restricted code is simpler, involves short, sharp exchanges, deals with practical matters, and is tied to the immediate context of the conversation. The meanings of the communications made with this code are often implicit. There is the assumption that the listener will know what is being talked about and little effort is made to provide what might appear to the speaker to be superfluous description. As the term implies, the elaborated code is more explanatory, complex and abstract. With the elaborated code there is a more explicit verbalisation of the meanings that the user of the restricted code takes for granted.

Critics of Bernstein's work have challenged his view that the restricted code is simpler than the elaborated code, and the implication that it is in some way inferior (Labov 1978). It is suggested that the language of the working class is as subtle as that of the middle class, but with different grammatical rules.

Furthermore, individuals may adopt both types of code depending on the circumstances. When two old friends meet, who have known each other since childhood, they use a restricted code because certain gestures or phrases 'speak a thousand words'. But when each is in a more formal environment they will use the elaborated code because of the need to explain concepts and ideas to unfamiliar people. Moreover, in post-modern society individuals may 'pick-and-mix' from various language codes in order to substantiate a lifestyle choice. Language in this sense therefore becomes yet another commodity.

Individuals are genetically endowed with male or female physical characteristics, but how they behave as men and women is largely socially prescribed. Studies of male and female behaviour in divergent cultural settings provide evidence to suggest that, to a significant extent, being a man or a woman is a social role. This view is supported by many anthropological studies of preindustrial, industrial and postindustrial societies. As Helman (1990) has reported, researchers have discovered a great variety of behaviour classified as appropriate for men and women.

Every society has its own set of acceptable patterns of behaviour or norms for the role of male and female. Language often demonstrates what is considered to be 'natural' behaviour for these roles. Lakoff (1975) discovered that in conversation men tended to be direct and assertive, whereas women were overpolite and passive.

As Hogg and Abrams (1988) have noted, there have also been changes in the more obvious ways in which language is used to differentiate between the two genders. Chairmen are now chairpersons, mankind has been renamed humanity and househusbands exist alongside housewives. Whether these changes are substantial or superficial remains questionable. Expectations of what is considered to be an appropriate way of behaving for a man or for a woman may not have altered fundamentally.

In Western societies women wear trousers, may decide not to have babies and live without male partners, and most gain paid employment. Men use facial moisturiser, may at some future date be able to have babies, and become nurses. There are also transgendered people who generate a considerable re-evaluation of conventional understandings of sexual identity. But, there has also been, for example, a resurgence of traditional 'masculinity' by men's movements (Giddens 2001), and research indicates that women remain tied to childcare and household responsibilities (Macionis & Plummer 1998). Moreover, Tannen (1992) has argued that men and women continue to speak different dialects, which she terms 'genderlects'. Communication, for Tannen, between men and women is as hampered as communication would be between two people from different cultures. The genderlect of men remains based on notions of independence and status, whereas that of women is based on connection and intimacy.

Men's talk frequently involves overt and covert references to the importance in personal and working relationships of maintaining their freedom to choose what they want to do, and of achieving high prestige. On the other hand, women regard it of greater importance to formulate close personal alliances with colleagues, family and friends. However, in situations where men and women are together in mixed-gender team meetings or classrooms, the male genderlect tends to dominate as this is perceived to be the norm by both men and women.

The research into gender and language has important implications for the way in which nurses communicate with service users and other health care professionals. This research suggests that female nurses persistently and unavoidably 'miscommunicate' with male patients, and male nurses 'miscommunicate' with female patients.

The majority of nurses are women, and therefore the occupation of nursing has a communicative bias towards a female genderlect. This, along with other reasons such as the medical professions' tactic of using new scientific discoveries as 'ideological ammunition' to maintain its relevant high status, may continue to prohibit the full professional emancipation of nursing (Morrall 2001). Whilst nursing communicates passivity, connection and intimacy, the male-dominated profession of medicine may maintain its superior position in the hierarchy of health care professions by communicating assertively its own high esteem, and the right to be autonomous in clinical practice.

Coates (1998), supported by a multitude of cross-cultural research studies, points out that it is the way men speak (i.e. the male genderlect) that is valued higher in all known societies. Moreover, challenging the stereotype that women are 'chatterboxes', research conducted in a variety of mixed-gender situations (for example, at work, and in school) demonstrates that men talk more than women do. Conversely, the stereotypical idea that women are universally more polite than men has some supportive evidence (Brown 1998). It is also incontrovertible that both women and men 'gossip', and that although the strategies used are not the same, each is attempting to achieve the outcome of increased group solidarity (Pilkington 1998).

However, language-use cannot be distinguished simply on the basis of gender because other social variables (for example, social class, age, and geographical region) affect linguistic style (Eckert 1998). This may mean that a female white middle-class and middle-aged senior executive of a financial centre in the City of London has more communication comparability to a man with a similar social status than a young black unemployed woman living in an impoverished area of Liverpool. Furthermore, social structure cuts across cultures and hence women (or men) based in the same structural position in different parts of the world may have communicative patterns that are alike:

... we would not expect linguistic similarities between West African women or high-caste Indian women and Tenejapan women, the former apparently having much more

structural power. But we can predict similarities between language usage of Tenejapan women [a community of Mayan Indians in Mexico] and other peasant women in egalitarian small-scale societies with similar social-structural features. (Brown, 1998, p. 97)

But, humans can make choices about what and how they want to communicate (Romaine 2000). Despite the prevailing social conditions that configure communication content and patterns, the female may decide consciously the linguistic style of someone outside either her local or wider cultural environment. Nurses communicating with patients may deliberately alter their speech code and the nonverbal signs they emit to achieve a premeditated objective. For example, a nurse working in an Accident and Emergency Department may want to gain information from a child about what poison, and how much of it, has been swallowed. Verbal and nonverbal communications (perhaps a smile, a touch, a soft-spoken voice, elementary words and phrases said with persistence but without causing unnecessary distress) will be adapted to suit this critical situation. An inexperienced junior doctor demanding immediate information on a medical ward about a patient's condition from the experienced Nurse-in-charge is likely to receive a contrasting but equally calculated communication.

Activity 3.4 The use of linguistic codes

Describe the type of linguistic 'code' used by you, your friends, your peers, other health care professionals, and health service users you come into contact with. Do you change your code depending upon with whom you are communicating?

DRAMA

One way of trying to comprehend the effects of the social context on communication is to view all interactions between human beings as representing a stageplay or drama. That is, what we say and do to each other are part of a scripted performance. Each actor adopts one or more roles during any performance. Tajfel and Fraser (1978) have defined 'role' as the required behaviour of someone in a given position, the term 'role performance' refers to the actual behaviour of the incumbent.

Entering into a clinical situation is similar to being an actor in a play, where service users, doctors and nurses are the actors in the cast. When interacting with a patient, communications are organised through the medium of the social role of a 'nurse' and communications are affected by the socially prescribed expectations of that role. Equally, the patient is communicating through his/her socially prescribed identity as a 'patient'.

Examples of the roles that may be enacted during any one day include possibly that of student nurse, son or daughter, brother or sister, friend and member of a sports team (Fig. 3.3). Each role serves as a social template, which fashions both what is sent by the communicator and what the other person receives. However, the way people behave in these roles will depend partly on how others behave towards them. If a student nurse is treated as subservient to doctors and senior nurses then the script will be different to that followed if he/she is treated as an adult by his/her personal tutor.

To follow the rules of a particular role, people need to know how others in associated roles behave. Hospital patients require information about the performances of the 'actors' they are going to meet in that institutional setting, for example, the nurses, doctors, physiotherapists, ward clerks and cleaners. For any role to exist, others must be executing their associated roles. An individual cannot be a student nurse unless there are qualified nurses, nurse lecturers and patients.

This theory of 'dramaturgy' has been advanced by, amongst others, Erving Goffman (1959). Goffman's idea was that society produced scripts, that is the guidelines for the performance of a role. These scripts were internalised by people through experience and the process of socialisation, enabling them to know how to behave in different circumstances.

Macionis and Plummer (1998) explain the drama of the doctor's surgery:

Consider, for example, how a doctor's surgery coveys information to an audience of patients. Doctors [still] enjoy prestige and power, a fact immediately grasped by patients upon entering the surgery or health centre. First, the doctor is nowhere to be seen. Instead, in what Goffman describes as the 'front region' of the setting, the patient encounters a receptionist who functions as a gatekeeper, deciding if and when the patient can meet the doctor. The doctor's private examination room of the surgery constitutes the 'back region' or the setting. Here the patient confronts a wide range of props, such as medical books and framed degrees, which together reinforce the impression that the doctor has the specialised knowledge to be in charge. In the surgery the

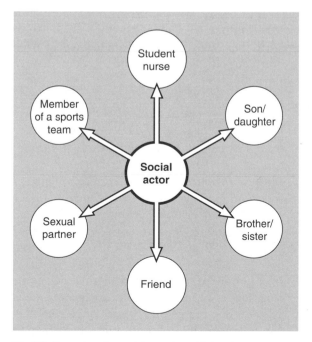

Fig 3.3 Examples of a social actor's multiple roles

doctor usually remains seated behind a desk – the larger the grander the desk, the greater the statement of power – while the patient is only provided with a chair. (Macionis & Plummer 1998, p. 162)

Macionis and Plummer (1998), again using Goffman's concept of role performance, provide another example of how doctors convey messages concerning their social status and motives for their chosen occupation. The ward-round, suggest Macionis and Plummer, becomes a staged event though which the illusion of in-depth knowledge of the patient (his/her medical condition and as an individual) can be communicated by the consultant to all of the other actors (i.e. the junior doctors, nurses and paramedical staff, and the relevant patient, and other patients who are observing the play). The consultant regimentally moves the multidisciplinary team around the stage to the end of a patient's bed), examines the medical notes, asks for information and suggestions from the entourage, and then sagely allows a tightly controlled 'audience-participation' interlude with the patient. Finally, the lead-actor moves off to re-enact a similar drama at another proscenium. The hospital is a theatre, however, that has many understudies for the (medical) lead-actors. Often it is the nurse, sometimes the physiotherapist or occupational therapist.

Scripts for social behaviour are regulated by specific rules that apply to the individual's particular circumstances. These rules predict how nurses will act when they are in the lecture theatre, on the ward, or at a dance. Problems arise when an individual enters a new situation and doesn't know the rules. However, general patterns of behaviour from previous experiences will suggest what actions might be normal and acceptable.

Student nurses may have faced, and be expected to face continuously, many novel and anxiety-provoking situations, for example, the first day in college or a new clinical experience. It may be considered important to get the rules of communication right in all social situations and particularly when meeting lecturers, other students, or colleagues for the first time. There will be a constant search for

the right thing to say and the appropriate gestures to make, combined with the recognition of social space and the necessary use of eye contact. Getting it wrong can cause lasting embarrassment. That is why some individuals try not to communicate too much, either verbally or nonverbally, until they have discovered what the rules are.

Just as student nurses have to sort out what to do in new situations, service users entering into hospital as inpatients or outpatients have to establish what the appropriate behaviour is in their role as patient. They have to find out what the organisational and interpersonal rules are, and this adds to the concerns they will already have for their clinical condition. A service user who is told that she has a major illness or disability may have to reconstitute many of her former role behaviours. Someone who has to have a leg amputated may not be able to perform her previous role at work or leisure.

In practice, roles cannot easily be compartmentalised as they have elaborate interconnections with each other. Some of the behaviour demonstrated in the role of friend may be replicated in the role of nurse. Although some of the behaviour expected in one role might be complementary to another there may be circumstances when roles are in tension. Abraham and Shanley (1992) explained:

As we move from one situation to another we may occupy the roles of nurse, club secretary, team member, mother, daughter, and political campaigner. The demands of these roles compete for our time and energy, leading to role conflict. A typical source of such role conflict is between obligations to family members and to those at work. (Abraham & Shanley, 1992, p. 76)

In addition to the conflict arising when the expectations of the different roles are incompatible, there are a number of other types of role conflict (Tajfel & Fraser 1978). For example, there may be disagreement amongst role occupants about the content of the role. Student nurses may have different views about what their role should be; some may study harder than others; some may view their role as 'just a job', whereas others may feel that nursing is a vocation (Mackay 1990). Individuals in other associated roles may disagree with the role occupant's interpretation of how to perform that role. Senior nurses perhaps have views about the way in which student nurses communicate with patients and other staff. These could be at variants to the views of the students themselves (Stockwell 1972).

Role conflict is managed through a number of different strategies. One example is where individuals distance themselves from one or more of their roles. Nursing is still regarded as essentially a female occupation. Therefore, the conflict between the gender and occupational identity of a male student nurse may be diffused by him joking about his role, or by stating that he intends to eventually become an educationalist or a manager.

Role conflict may lead to what Ebaugh (1988) described as 'role exit'. The person decides to stop adhering to a particular role, for example leave his/her employment, or separate from a partner. However, some roles (for example, that of father, mother, son and daughter) cannot be easily exited if at all. They are (usually) lifelong performances. Moreover, roles that involve a high degree of what Goffman (1959) described as 'spoiled identity' may be extremely difficult to shake off. That is, the person's self-understanding is contaminated by the (usually) negative consequences of a label given by others. For example, it may be that if someone has been in the care of the mental health services or has suffered a life-threatening cancer, but is no longer receiving treatment, he/she is classified by the preceding label. He/she is an 'ex'-mental patient or 'in remission', or 'a 5-year cancer survivor'. It is the way in which verbal, nonverbal, and written communications by health care professionals are constituted on the basis of the previous health problem that perpetuates the spoiled identity. For example, whenever he or she comes into contact with the health service then the medical history will dictate to some degree the style and content of the interaction. In Foucault's (1973) terms, the 'medical gaze' will focus on signs of madness or physical debilitation.

Activity 3.5 An exercise in social identity

Examine your reactions to the next three people you meet. Apart from what was stated verbally, what 'hidden' messages were being transmitted by you and by them about your respective status, age, social class, and gender?

MEDIA

McLuhan's (1964) insightful dictum that 'the media is the message' testifies to the mode of communication tending to configure the meaning and importance of what is being transmitted.

Electronic media disgorge information to such an extent and concerning so many issues, that it can be argued a worldwide single culture is disseminated, thereby forging a 'global village' (McLuhan 1964). Human communication is becoming increasingly mediated by electronic devices (Schultz 2001).

The consequences of 'mass communication' for interpersonal communication are dynamic if debatable. In the electronically connected and global village, images and actualities of shared but diverse social realities are transmitted via the Internet, video, film and television. With reference to health care, self-help information and groups abound on the Internet, and there is now in the UK an electronic consultation system within the National Health Service, 'NHS Direct' operated, in the main, by nurses.

The perpetual visual and aural outpourings of television is, however, particularly effective in penetrating our interpersonal communication. Television (especially digital and cable) bombards the viewers with special types of information. These are special in the sense that they have the effect of producing a set of values and themes that configure our understanding of the world in our immediate vicinity, and also construe our impression of distant lands. We travel the world from our settees and internalise the visited cultures (which have already been swayed by the economic and political exigencies of globalisation). Individuals become so affected by what is seen and heard via television that their very self-identity is formulated by its content (Barker 1999). We talk habitually about programmes we have watched, and along with the weather and public transport, talk about television acts as the 'social glue' of conversation. Significantly, television characters, fictional or real, become 'models' for our behaviour. Emulated or despised, these characters are insidiously incarnated within our own personalities.

However, the written word has not been supplanted by electronic signals. Literary output is prolific and worldwide in the form of books, newspapers and magazines. Moreover, script is an integral ingredient of the most flourishing type of electronic communication – the email and the text message. There are now trillions of words zooming around the communicative medium of cyberspace. Face-to-face interpersonal communication is being relocated to cyberspace, pulsating along the electronic gadgetry of the Internet and mobile phones.

Taking McLuhan's stance that the medium is the message, the computer and its web of communicative accessories may be accused of fashioning our thoughts and abilities to express those thoughts if only because of the (to-date) discrepancy between physiology and electronics. Humans do not transmit messages to each other when in close proximity in the same way as they do when typing and sending a message to a loved-one, friend or colleague, twenty thousand kilometres away even if the dialogue is in real-time. More interestingly and alarmingly, humans lose their corporeality within cyberspace. They become the message on the screen. Their world is amorphous, taking any shape and size depending on their imaginations and intentions rather than physical boundaries. The consequences can be social isolation, whereby contact with other humans is reduced, and a blurring of working and personal lives (Giddens 2001).

Mobile phones, alongside the Internet, have had an enormous impact on interpersonal communication. In the 10 years leading up to the new millennium, the number of mobile phones in use throughout the world accelerated at an astonishing rate – from 11 million in 1990 to 400 million in 2000 (Giddens 2001). On the positive side, mobile phones offer an immediate and accessible means of personal communication. On the negative side, they supplant face-to-face communication, and also their operation in public situations (for example, restaurants, bars and trains) interferes with the personal space of others.

Moreover, 'personal space' has become intermeshed with the communicative outpourings of 'social space' when using the Internet. That is, using McQuail's 'Pyramid of Communication' (see above), dialogue at the intrapersonal and interpersonal levels enters the group, organisation, society-wide and global levels whenever we send material to multiple-user websites. Our ideas are exposed to an extensive audience. Furthermore, governments have become more keen to 'spy' on Internet communications following the attack on the 'Twin Towers' in New York (during the now notorious day of September the 11th 2001) so that terrorist interchanges can be intercepted. Such prying, no matter how necessary, results in a significant dilution of private communication.

Jean Baudrillard (1995) has described how contemporary mass media (especially television) assist in defining our world, rather than merely representing that world, to a degree that even such apparently uncontestable events as war are 'made-up'. Events (perhaps all of social life) are contrived, illusions, in the sense that they take place via, but also for, television. But not only are they shown on television, each incident within the event is conveyed to a worldwide audience. The audience (including those supposedly in charge of the event – in the case of a war, the generals and political leaders) has to be entertained and/or informed, and therefore incidents are intermingled with actual happenings and media narrative and imagery. This intermingling of fact and media-fiction manufactures a 'hyperreality'. Consequently, interpersonal communication is not just 'distorted', as Habermas (1970, 1972) has suggested, by the requirements of capitalism, but by the very particular needs of the media. We watched the destruction of the Twin Towers in New York and the armed conflict in Afghanistan 'live'. Here we had television spectacles in which heroes and villains were moulded by news reporters and the television programme editors in front of our eyes.

However, both Baudrillard and Habermas can be reproached for regarding the audience, that is all of us, as too quiescent. Thompson (1995) has argued that humans could be judicious in how they interpret media narrative and imagery. Although interpersonal communication is affected by what stories those running the media decide to broadcast, and mechanism of distribution, people talk with others about these stories, decipher and assign their own meanings to the events. For example, the media may portray diseases such as AIDS, measles, skin cancer, or influenza, as highly dangerous and a threat to all or certain sections of society (perhaps young heterosexuals, children, holidaymakers or the elderly). However, this does not mean that everyone, or all of those in the vulnerable groups, will adopt precautionary measures. Through intrapersonal and interpersonal critical discussion, some people will challenge these messages, and consciously ignore what they may decide is media 'hype'. Steven Miles (2001) has suggested that people are not slaves of popular culture (which includes the media). People think and make judgements about even such prominent social edifices as television.

However, Schultz (2001) has argued that 'distance communication' is not necessarily qualitatively different to face-to-face communication. That is, it is not inevitable that talking with someone who is sitting beside you means that there is better understanding taking place. For example, the social surroundings of a discussion between a senior nurse and student nurse about a particular clinical procedure that has to be carried out may be affected detrimentally by preconceived views about the other's identity (for example, ethnic group, gender or age). Communication via email, Internet discussion sites or the telephone (mobile and landline), whilst losing nonverbal clues, has the advantage of 'hiding' the social status of the participants and therefore becomes more egalitarian. For Schultz (2001), there is a potential richness in distance communication that tends to be ignored.

Schultz points out that theorising and research to-date into distance communication has tended to accept the idea that those involved become 'virtual entities' rather than 'real entities'. That is, the lack of contextual clues about the other person results in him/her becoming something other than an embodied creature with a recognisable physical shape and personality during computerised discussion. We conjure-up an appearance and psychological disposition for the other 'thing', which may bear no relation to the authentic person. Moreover, the participants may deliberately misrepresent themselves, for example, claiming to be a different gender or age.

However, rather than virtual communication being a separate mode of social intercourse to that of real communication, there are many interconnections. For example, 'the presentation of self in every day life' (to use Goffman's phrase, 1959) is a dynamic process even without the introduction of electronic communication. Although our self-identity is insidiously and continuously influenced by the reactions of others, we also conspire to offer certain aspects or our 'selves' to others and conceal other elements.

Activity 3.6 Health messages in the media

Review four episodes of different television soap operas and six national newspapers (three tabloid and three broadsheet), identifying issues relating to health. What are the messages being communicated about health in these media? Are these messages consistent or are there inconsistencies?

CONCLUSION

Health care professionals are in an occupation that has interpersonal communication at its very core. Virtually all nursing work revolves around the need for nurses to be effective communicators, whether relating to colleagues or with service users. This is indicated in the content of contemporary educational programmes. Although the subject of interpersonal communication now receives considerable attention from nurse educators, it is of limited value to examine communication only at the level of the overt verbal and nonverbal messages.

When reflecting upon acts of interpersonal communication there is a requirement to consider the wider social context, the social characteristics of the sender and receiver of the communication, and the structure of the power relationships between those involved. There is a necessity for nurses to become sensitive to how their communications are influenced and distorted by social factors before accurate communication, or what Habermas (1970, 1972) has described as 'communicative competency', can be achieved.

Taking into account these social factors the next time you are asked in a bar or café, 'Hello, how are you?' (or you ask this of a health service user), may increase your interpersonal communicative competency.

REFERENCES

Abraham C, Shanley E 1992 Social psychology for nurses. Edward Arnold, London

Armstrong D 1984 The patient's view. Social Science and Medicine 18(9): 737–744

Barker C 1999 Television, globalization and cultural identities. Open University Press, Buckingham

Baudrillard J 1995 The Gulf War did not take place. Power Publications, Sydney

Bernstein B 1975 Class, codes and control. Routledge & Kegan Paul, London

Boseley S 2001 Patients are often left in the dark, admit surgeons. The Guardian 8th November

Brooks P 1993 Body works: objects of desire in modern narrative. Harvard University Press, Harvard

Brown P 1998 How and why are women more polite: Some evidence from a Mayan community. In: Coates J (ed) Language and gender: a reader, Ch 7, pp 81–91. Blackwell, Oxford

Coates J (ed) 1998 Language and gender: a reader. Blackwell, Oxford

Collins BE, Raven BH 1969 Group structure: attraction, coalitions, communication and power. In: Lindzey G, Aronson E (eds) The handbook of social psychology, Vol. 4, 2nd edn. Addison-Wesley, Reading, MA

Crook S, Pakulski J, Waters M 1992 Postmodernisation: change in advanced society. Sage, London

Dowding K 1996 Power. Open University Press, Buckingham

Ebaugh H 1988 Becoming an EX: The process of role exit. University of Chicago Press, Chicago

Eckert P 1998 Gender and sociolinguistic variation. In: Coates J (ed) Language and gender: a reader, Ch 6, pp 64–80. Blackwell, Oxford

Foucault M 1971 Madness and civilisation. Tavistock, London

Foucault M 1973 The birth of the clinic. Tavistock, London

Foucault M 1974 The order of things. Tavistock, London

Foucault M 1980 Power/knowledge, selected interviews and other writings 1972–1977. Harvester, Brighton

Freidson 1970 The profession of medicine: A study of applied sociology of knowledge. Dodd Mead, New York

French JRP, Raven BH 1959 The bases of social power. In: Cartwright D (ed) Studies in social power. University of Michigan Press, Michigan

Giddens A 1984 The constitution of society. Polity Press, Cambridge

Giddens A 1991 Modernity and self-identity: Self and society in the late modern age. Polity Press, Cambridge

Giddens A 2001 Sociology, 4th edn. Polity Press, Cambridge

Goffman E 1959 The presentation of self in everyday life. Penguin, Harmondsworth

Gumperz J 1968 The speech community. International encyclopedia of the social sciences, 2nd edn. Macmillan, London

Habermas J 1970 Towards a rational society. Heinemann, London

Habermas J 1972 Knowledge and human interests. Heinemann, London

Hartley P 1993 Interpersonal communication. Routledge, London

Helman CG 1990 Culture, health and illness, 2nd edn. Wright, London

Hogg MA, Abrams D 1988 Social identifications. Routledge, London

Hugman R 1991 Power in caring professions. Macmillan, Basingstoke

Labov W 1978 Sociolinguistic patterns. Blackwell, Oxford

Lakoff R 1975 Language and a woman's place. Harper and Row, New York

Laurance J 2002 Doctors want nurses to become NHS 'gate-keepers'. The Independent 28th February

Macionis J, Plummer K 1998 Sociology: a global introduction. Prentice Hall, London

Mackay L 1990 Nursing: just another job? In: Abbott P, Wallace W (eds) The sociology of the caring professions. Falmer, London

McKie R 2001 Revealed: the secret of human behaviour. The Observer 11th February

McLuhan M 1964 Understanding media. Routledge and Kegan Paul, London

McQuail D 1984 Communication, 2nd edn. Longman, Harlow

McQuail D 2000 McQuail's mass communication theory, 4th edn. Sage, London

Malhotra VA 1987 Habermas' sociological theory as a basis for clinical practice with small groups. Clinical Sociology Review 5: 181–192

Miller DC, Form WH 1962 Industrial sociology. Harper and Row, London

Miles S 2001 Social theory in the real world. Sage, London

Morrall PA 2001 Sociology and nursing. Routledge, London

Parsons T 1951 The social system. Routledge & Kegan Paul, London

Pilkington J 1998 'Don't try to make out that I'm nice!' The different strategies women and men use when gossiping. In: Coates J (ed) Language and gender: a reader, Ch 17, pp 254–269. Blackwell, Oxford

Romaine S 2000 Language in society: an introduction to sociolinguistics, 2nd edn. Oxford University Press, Oxford

Schatzman L, Strauss A 1955 Social class and modes of communication. American Journal of Sociology 60(4): 329–338

Schultz T 2001 Distance communication. Zeitschrift Fur Soziologie 30(2): 85–102

Stockwell F 1972 The unpopular patient: the study of nursing care reports. Series 1, No. 2. Royal College of Nursing, London

Szasz T, Hollender MH 1956 A contribution to the philosophy of medicine. American Medical Association's Archives of Internal Medicine XCVII: 585–592

Tajfel H, Fraser C 1978 Introducing social psychology. Penguin, Harmondsworth

Tannen D 1992 You just don't understand: women and men in conversation. Virago, London

Thompson J 1995 The media and modernity: a social theory of the media. Polity Press, Cambridge

Wolpert L 2002 It wasn't me, it was my genes. The Independent, 15th February

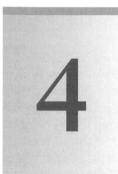

Psychological factors affecting communication

Stuart A. Hindle

INTRODUCTION

In Chapter 1, the differences between inter- and intrapersonal communication were described. In practice, they interact with each other in subtle ways.

This chapter will explore those differences and introduce the concept of communication filters and the ways in which context influences communication.

Also discussed will be developmental factors and the application of concepts to the following client groups:

◆ the child;
◆ the mentally ill;
◆ the person with learning disabilities;
◆ the elderly.

DEVELOPMENTAL FACTORS AFFECTING COMMUNICATION

Nature versus nurture

Communication is a complex process involving both interpersonal and intrapersonal factors. Each person is a unique individual, with a unique interpretation of the world, influenced by origin, upbringing and life experience.

Is an individual's personality shaped by genetic, hereditary factors (nature), or is it shaped by the environment in which he lives (nurture)? Most Schools of Psychology offer arguments in favour of one approach or the other, although some may believe both to be important (see Box 4.1).

Box 4.1 Nature or nurture?

1. The biological approach favours nature and believes it to comprise of biological systems which are only partially influenced by the environment.

2. The behaviourist approach stresses the effect of the environment and persons within it as the source of reward and punishment. It is therefore on the side of nurture.

3. The cognitive approach suggests that the debate about nature versus nurture is irrelevant. Both have equal input into the way an individual perceives the world.

4. The humanist approach of Rogers and Maslow emphasises that nature and nurture are merely boundaries within which human nature is free to develop its full potential.

5. The psychodynamic approach reinforces the impact of the effects of the environment upon the unconscious behaviour of the person.

With the recent development of the science of Genetics and the Human Genome Project, it is now possible to identify genes for specific bodily functions and hence determine the cause of many genetic disorders.

Geneticists are also stating that every aspect of human functioning, including behaviour, could be determined by our genes.

In the deepest sense we are who we are because of our genes (Robert Sinsheimer 1991)

Sir James Watson the co-discoverer of the structure of DNA stated:

Now we know, in large measure, our fate is in our genes (Jaroff 1989)

Many researchers have attributed genetic causes to behavioural disorders such as schizophrenia, alcoholism and manic depression. However, in several cases, these assertions have either been modified or retracted. For a discussion of this in relation to alcoholism see Peele (1990) and Couzigou et al (1999).

This debate does raise the spectre of eugenics which is the science of improving the human race by selective breeding, popular with the Nazis in 1940s. During the 1970s in the USA, Dr Arnold Hutschnecker proposed that all American children be psychologically tested at age six with inkblots to determine criminal tendencies. These 'future delinquents' would then be sent off to appropriate 'camps' where they would learn more socially acceptable behaviour patterns.

Another aspect of the nature versus nurture debate is how much of human nature is predestined, and how much is free will? This has led people to say 'I'm fat because it's in my genes'.

Research has been carried out into this question particularly with monozygotic twins who develop from the same egg, but are raised apart. To date around 300 studies have been carried out worldwide and many pairs of twins do exhibit very similar behavioural traits.

Critics of this type of research have pointed out that often twins in these studies were raised by relatives or close family friends and, in some cases, the twins made contact with each other as they were growing up.

It would seem that there is no absolute answer to the question of whether the individual is a product of their genes or their upbringing, it is more a question of to what extent are optimum environments created for innate tendencies to be fully expressed?

What seems certain is the lack of simple conclusive answers to describe the uniqueness of the individual, although some factors, particularly internal ones, can be described. For example:

◆ defence mechanisms;
◆ attitudes;
◆ assumptions;
◆ prejudices;
◆ perceptual distortions.

These factors modify external stimuli and determine the way in which a person will respond to them. The physical and cultural contexts of the interaction are also important. These will be discussed later in the chapter.

Activity 4.1 gives you an opportunity to explore your own perceptions of the influences of nature and nurture.

Activity 4.1 Nature versus nurture

Write down a list of things which attracted you to nursing. Underline those which you feel were to do with your inner value system and beliefs and circle those which you feel were influenced by others. When you look through the list again you may notice that some of the factors you underlined in the first instance may have actually been influenced by others in the past and have become integrated into your value system.

COGNITIVE DEVELOPMENT

Before going on to discuss interpersonal aspects of communication it would be useful to briefly summarize theories on how children develop cognitively from birth through to adolescence.

Children are not 'little adults'. They have a different perception of the world based upon their stage of development and individual experiences.

The most influential theorist in the area of child development was Jean Piaget (1896–1980). He described four major developmental stages which a child went through. These are:

1. 0–2 years. The sensorimotor stage when babies are only aware of things in the environment which impact upon their senses directly. They are always experimenting to learn by trial and error, usually by putting things in their mouth or throwing them away.

2. 2–7 years. The preoperational stage where children think about things in symbolic terms. They can pretend, understand past and future, but

comparison, cause and effect are still not possible. A classic experiment at this stage was to pour all the water from a tall, thin jar into a short, fat one in front of the child and then ask them which glass held the most fluid. Piaget found that children at this age said that it was the tall, thin jar which held the most. This illustrated that children of this age were unable to 'conserve' (Piaget & Inhelder 1969).

3. 7–12 years. The concrete operational stage where the child can now cope with conservation, understanding numbers, reversibility and some problem solving. They are now aware of events outside of their lives. Thought patterns are still not abstract and logic is still not fully developed.

4. 12 years and above. The formal operations stage where there is more formal logic and abstract thought. Children are able to think systematically, make deductions and develop their own values, beliefs and philosophies.

There have been criticisms of Piaget's theories more recently. Piaget based most of his conclusions upon observing the behaviour of his own three children, a very small unreliable sample.

Flanagan (1996) cites other criticisms of Piaget's findings such as some of his experiments not making any sense. In the conservation experiments, Piaget asked the children the same question before and after the transformation. A younger child may think that there should be a different answer to the second question. This experiment has been repeated whereby the experimenter only asked the conservation question after the transformation had taken place. Many younger children were able to conserve. See also Bremmer and Bryant (2001) for an account of a repeat experiment on the effect of spatial cues on infant's responses with and without a hidden object.

Other theorists who describe child development view it from their own background. So there are biological theories as discussed in the previous section, social learning theories which stem from behaviourism and psychodynamic theories which emphasise the unconscious motivations influencing development. For a more detailed discussion of these approaches see Lindon (1998).

THE INTER/ INTRAPERSONAL MIX

Human communication is a highly complex activity of interaction involving others as well as oneself. What one person intends in the interaction is not always understood by the other person. Consider the example given in Box 4.2.

Box 4.2 shows how, on the surface, it would seem that information had been given from one person to another in a quiet room with no apparent distractions. The Oxford Dictionary (1998) describes communication as 'something that communicates information from one person to another'. However, this does not take account of the complex interpersonal and extrapersonal factors that are involved.

In the example given in Box 4.2, Sarah was anxious about meeting new people in a new setting and her bladder was becoming increasingly uncomfortable. The terms used by lecturers to describe the course were unfamiliar to Sarah, and were forgotten almost immediately. There were certain communication filters involved that blocked or distorted the message sent from the lecturers. These filters will be explored later in the chapter.

Several authors have attempted to devise a model of the intrapersonal factors involved in communication episodes (Pluckman 1978, Hargie 1997). These are summarised in Figure 4.1.

In this process, the sense organs receive stimuli. The nervous system then perceives these stimuli, processing them into symbols that are then checked with those already stored in the memory. This is the point at which all a person's past experiences, attitudes, beliefs and values influence what happens next. If there is consistency between what is perceived and all these factors, then meaning is generated and a response occurs. However, if as in Sarah's case, there is an incongruity because of her lack of understanding

---

Box 4.2 The interaction of inter- and intrapersonal factors

Sarah Jones arrived for her first day on the Diploma in Nursing course at the local University. She was anxious about meeting new people and her bladder was feeling full. She had expectations of the course lecturers that were based on her perceptions of teachers from her school days 15 years ago.

The other students looked so bright and confident, Sarah was sure they would have no trouble on the course. The lecturers introduced themselves and gave a brief talk about the course: its structure, the assessment strategy and the competencies to be achieved.

After 30 minutes, the lecturers felt satisfied that they had introduced themselves and given an overview on the course. Sarah on the other hand was confused – she did not yet know any of the other students and felt her bladder was about to burst.

---

and an overriding need to find the toilet, then meaning will be lost.

Maslow (1954) pointed out in his human needs hierarchy, that unless basic physiological needs are met (including the need to empty the bladder) little else will be of importance. In the example given, had teaching staff offered beverages before the introduction, pointed out where the toilets were, and asked for any questions, the intrapersonal conflict that occurred could have been at least partially resolved. Teaching staff had obviously been through the process of introducing students to the course on several occasions and because they were no longer sensitive to the technical language, they assumed that the students had the same level of understanding.

Unfortunately this is a trap into which many professionals fall. Medical and nursing staff become so accustomed to using technical language with each other that when they give information to patients, it too becomes loaded with jargon.

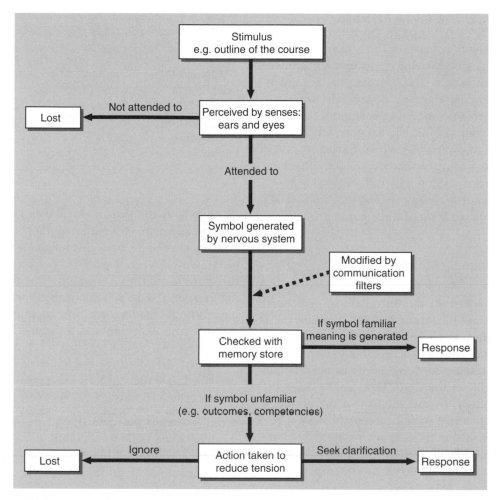

Fig 4.1 A model of intrapersonal communication

It is important, therefore, for nurses to communicate with patients at an appropriate level of understanding, as outlined in Chapter 5.

COMMUNICATION FILTERS

Communication filters were often referred to in earlier texts as barriers. However, this word would seem to indicate that they create a complete block to incoming information. In reality, the information is distorted or filtered rather than blocked. There are many possible factors that may act as

---

Box 4.3 Communication filters

Defence mechanisms
Attitudes, beliefs and values
Attributions and assumptions
Prejudices
Perceptual distortions

---

filters to communication and the ones that commonly occur are listed in Box 4.3 and are described in more detail below.

DEFENCE MECHANISMS

When a person behaves in an unexpected way, usually displaying extreme emotions such as anger or sorrow, it is said that 'his defences are down' or 'he is showing his true colours'. The 'defences' referred to are unconscious mechanisms described by Anna Freud (1946), the daughter of Sigmund Freud. Everyday phrases such as 'having repressed feelings' or 'having a fixation' about something are taken from psychoanalytical terminology.

According to Freud's theory an individual's personality is made up of three parts:

◆ the id;
◆ the ego;
◆ the superego.

The id represents the unconscious, instinctual desires that are unrestrained – self gratification is the goal. However, when interacting with others, it is not always socially acceptable to satisfy one's desires. A restraining force needs to operate and this is the role of the 'ego'. The 'ego' modifies the instinctual urges of the 'id' so that the person is able to interact in a socially acceptable way.

However, within these structures there is still no moral code, no guilt or shame. The third structure that achieves this is known as the 'superego' or conscience.

The development of these three components of the personality can be seen in a child from infancy to about 4 years of age, according to Sigmund Freud (1954). The infant reacts with basic instinctual drives and is completely self-centred. At around 2–3 years of age, the child begins to relate to others and modifies his desires according to the reinforcements he obtains from the parent, such as chastisement or praise.

As the child develops language, phrases such as 'Don't do that', 'Do as you are told' and 'It's naughty to hit your brother' impart a set of preferred behaviours to him. This learning and internalising of preferred behaviours is termed socialisation and can continue to develop and be modified throughout life.

Box 4.4 Common defence mechanisms
Rationalisation
Regression
Repression
Denial
Identification
Projection
Fantasy

As long as the person's wellbeing is intact, the ego and superego will work together to modify or hold in check the basic instinctual urges of the id. However, when a person's wellbeing is under threat, to avoid the id breaking through and causing irresponsible behaviour, or the superego breaking through leading to overwhelming feelings of guilt, the ego enlists defence mechanisms to counteract this.

Nearly 20 defence mechanisms have been described, but they all have the same characteristics according to Emslie (1979). These are that:

◆ self-esteem is maintained;
◆ anxiety and guilt are reduced;
◆ there is an indirect liberation of instinctual expression in an unconscious way.

Some of the more common defence mechanisms that have been described are listed in Box 4.4 and are described briefly below.

Rationalisation

Rationalisation occurs when an individual gives reasons for behaviour that, to the individual, seem perfectly reasonable. For example, a student states that he will start work on his essay as soon as he has watched the 'important' documentary on television.

Phrases such as 'I'll give up smoking as soon as I pass the exam' or the man who says 'the relationship was heading for the rocks anyway' as his girlfriend leaves are other examples where the person wants something to occur but can't achieve it.

The nurse, who having repeatedly ignored the patient's call buzzer because she doesn't like to talk to him, states 'I'm so busy with the care plans that I can't see to him now'.

Regression

Regression is characterised by behaviour appropriate to an earlier stage of development. Thumb sucking by an adult is a mild form of this. Bedwetting by an older child after a change in a familiar environment, such as going into hospital, is another example.

An extreme example occurs in some forms of mental illness such as depression when a patient may curl up in a corner in the fetal position, regressing back to the womb.

Repression

Repression is an unconscious submerging of memories and feelings by an individual, usually of past events, to avoid anxiety or guilt feelings.

The person who witnesses the results of a terrorist bomb attack, or is involved in an armed conflict may lose partial or total memory of the events. However, the memories are still there and can lead to physical symptoms such as tiredness and weakness.

Denial

Denial is an unconscious defence mechanism used by an individual against anxiety-inducing events, even in the face of such events. For example, loss of consciousness or fainting when receiving an emotional shock is a form of denial. Denial is seen most frequently when there is grief or severe loss, either of a person, or a body part such as amputation of a limb. The widow who sets the table at home for two and states 'Frank will be home soon from work. He always likes his tea on the table' is exhibiting a severe form of denial.

Identification

Identification is admiration of another person to the point of taking on some of the characteristics of that person. Usually, the person is famous and may be a film star, a sportsperson or a well known public figure. Some theorists believe that by identifying with a particular character on film, a sort of catharsis, or release of primitive instinctual urges takes place in a safe, controlled way.

Others dispute this however, by stating that the more a person is exposed to violence and sex on film or TV the more likely they are to take on these behaviours themselves. For a review of the research into this area see Glover (1985).

Projection

Projection occurs when a person's undesirable traits are attributed to, or projected upon, others to avoid punishment. Thus the person who has an unconscious prejudice against someone of another race, may project those feelings onto a second person, accusing them of being a bigot.

Fantasy

Fantasy is the use of the imagination to conjure up an image of something that is desired by an individual. Usually, the object or person is unobtainable. Most people engage in fantasy. It can be used as a means of stress reduction, such as imagining being on a beach in the sun with the rhythmic sound of the waves breaking on the shore. However, too much time spent in fantasy means that less time is spent in reality. This can lead to daydreaming and nonattentive behaviour, and is obviously undesirable where others are involved.

Defence mechanisms may have a short-term beneficial effect in maintaining self-esteem and reducing anxiety and guilt. However, if deployed inappropriately, they can cause severe distortions of reality in that they can affect the way an individual perceives and interacts with others.

ATTITUDES, BELIEFS AND VALUES

A person's beliefs and values strongly predict what attitude will be adopted to a particular event. An individual's attitude is observable by others in the form of behaviour, whereas beliefs and values are not.

According to Adler and Rodman (1991):

1. An attitude is a response to something in either a positive or a negative way.
2. A belief is a conviction of the right of something based on cultural upbringing.
3. A value is at the core of the person. It is a belief in the worth of a concept. Values are usually embodied in complex moral or religious systems that are found in all cultures and societies (Activity 4.2).

Activity 4.2 Attitudes, beliefs and values

In this activity think of your attitudes towards university, work, politics and sport. Make a statement about each area down one side of the page and on the other side list the people or groups that have influenced your attitude and the way in which they did this. Which attitudes were more difficult to describe in terms of their origin and why?

Attitudes, beliefs and values are acquired: a person is not born with them. Most fundamental beliefs and values are gained from those who influence the individual most – parents, siblings, teachers, friends and media figures.

Children are rewarded for displaying the 'right' attitude and punished for displaying the 'wrong' one. Eventually, through positive or negative reinforcement (see Chapter 2) the behaviour will either continue, or become extinguished.

Children also take on the behaviour or attitudes of role models by observation and imitation. Parents are amongst the most important role models, but television personalities or cartoon characters can also have a strong effect. Media use has been made of humour to encourage people to live a healthy lifestyle. According to Niven (2000), research on attitude formation shows that attitudes towards health are best influenced in the formative years and are more lasting. Therefore health education should start at an early age. Parents and the media are in an ideal position to achieve this.

It is through socialisation and interpersonal communication that people develop attitudes, beliefs and values. These in turn effect the unique way in which a person views the world. It is this uniqueness that acts as a filter to communication and can lead to misunderstanding and misinterpretation. People who have the same basic concept of something don't always believe in it the same way. For example, two people may express a belief that waste should be recycled, yet only one takes used paper and bottles to the waste banks.

Someone may hold a belief that smoking is a bad habit and yet continue to smoke. This can generate frustration and anger among health care staff when the patient is readmitted for a third time during winter suffering with chronic bronchitis.

Changing people's attitudes

Health professionals are involved daily in attempting to change people's attitudes. Knowledge of how attitudes are changed would therefore be useful. According to Kagan et al (1986) it is the need in most people to maintain consistency, that is the key to attitude change. Theorists state that attitudes have three components:

◆ a thinking component (cognitive);
◆ an emotional component (affective);
◆ an action component (conative).

Change occurring in any one of these three should bring about a change in the others. See the example in Box 4.5.

If the patient described in Box 4.5 is advised by health care staff, or other patients, that smoking

A man with heart disease may continue to smoke despite advice from all sources to give up. If this patient considered that smoking was hazardous, his attitude could be characterised by thoughts, feelings and actions that are consistent with each other.

'I think (cognition) that smoking is insignificant as a cause of my heart condition. I like smoking (affective). I will carry on smoking (conative).'

has a definite effect on heart disease, it will create inconsistency or tension within the system and there will be an attempt to reduce the habit. This state of tension is known as cognitive dissonance (Festinger 1957). When faced with this dilemma, several courses of action could take place.

The man could change his attitude towards smoking so that it is consistent with this new information. He could seek out new information that is consistent with his current attitude, such as reports of studies suggesting smoking has few or no ill effects. Or he could cite a relative who lived to 90 years of age and smoked all his life.

Lastly, the smoker could minimise or reduce the importance of the inconsistency by ignoring the leaflets or advice. 'It's the only pleasure I have in life. We all have to die from something'. Nurses therefore, may need to be particularly persuasive in their attempts to change attitudes.

Persuasive messages

According to Niven (2000) there are three elements of persuasive messages:

◆ the characteristics of the communicator;
◆ the communication itself;
◆ the characteristics of the recipient.

The communicator

The communicator must be credible and a recognised expert. A first-year student nurse who states that regular exercise is important for physical wellbeing would have less impact than a consultant physician or a top sports personality.

The communication

The message may be emotional or fear inducing in which case the appeal should be strong. Individuals must believe that they are at risk if they ignore the message and that the danger will pass if they follow the advice.

The message may appeal to reason, whereby a one- or two-sided argument can be put forward. In the example of the smoker, a two-sided argument would probably work better, presenting the evidence from both perspectives and highlighting the flaws in the pro-smoking argument.

Use of appropriate humour is essential in making a message stick in the mind of a patient or client. This is evident in the field of advertising where annual awards are given to those judged the most humorous.

Methods of presenting information will influence groups or individuals in different ways. Some people will respond readily to visual communication of film or demonstration whilst others may prefer the written or spoken word.

The recipient

Kagan et al (1986) and Niven (2000) have discussed the characteristics of the recipient of the message. It was thought that people with a low self-esteem were more likely to be persuaded than those with a high self-esteem. However, more recently, cognitive arguments have been put forward. These claim that a person is less likely to change his mind if he is able to think of a number of counter-arguments to the message. Sometimes a person will go out of his way to do the opposite of what he has been told so as not to appear to have lost the right to think for himself.

For the health professional to deliver a persuasive message, it is necessary to have an awareness of how a person's attitudes, beliefs and values will influence the reception of that message. The professional's value system is not necessarily the same as that of the patient.

ATTRIBUTIONS AND ASSUMPTIONS

People often make assumptions about each other on very flimsy evidence, such as the type of clothing worn, style of speaking, and the role held in society.

A certain amount of labelling occurs as a result of such assumptions. For example, a man wearing a clerical collar will be labelled as religious, pious, a paragon of virtue, a comforter and counsellor. If these labels are reinforced enough by others, then the individual may begin to take on these characteristics in excess. This is known as a self-fulfilling prophecy (Activity 4.3).

Activity 4.3 Attributions and assumptions

List any changes in your behaviour since you became a student nurse on one side of a piece of paper. On the other side, explain why these changes have occurred. What does this say about labelling and the self-fulfilling prophecy?

Labelling can lead to stereotyping whereby people are slotted into neat pigeon-holes. This mechanism helps maintain consistency and when something occurs to change the label or stereotype, cognitive dissonance occurs.

The clergyman who is reported in the press as having an affair with one of his parishioners will immediately undergo a label change. The blame will be laid fully on him by an outraged public because he betrayed the stereotype of a typical clergyman.

The fault will lie with him rather than with some other external agency (i.e. the woman, his

wife, or the pressures of his job). Fritz Heider (1958) suggested that when observing behaviour, individuals attempt to use a cause and effect analysis to make sense of it. He described two types of cause:

◆ dispositional (personal);
◆ situational (environmental).

People tend to attribute dispositional causes to others when something goes wrong, and attribute situational causes to themselves. When one person sees another fall down the stairs, clumsiness may be seen as the cause. If, however, the same thing happens to the observer, a loose carpet may be blamed.

When attempting to account for behaviour, an individual is more apt to attribute negative behaviours to environmental factors and positive behaviours to personal factors. For example 'I was angry because the carpet was loose' or, 'He was so clumsy, I had to go and help him up'.

The problem with such assumptions is that in the case of the other person falling over, the situational factors such as a loose carpet, slippery shoes, or an object on the stairs is not taken into account; the context of the behaviour is ignored. This is known as attribution error. An area where attribution theory is reversed is in the case of clinical depression.

Rather than attribute negative behaviour to situational factors, the depressed person will blame himself. Positive behaviour is attributed to situational factors, often temporary, yet very specific, such as, 'I ate my breakfast today because it was a cereal I like.'

PREJUDICES

Prejudice involves making assumptions about people and attributing certain labels and stereotypes to them. Prejudice can be seen in many aspects of life, often in relation to:

◆ race;
◆ colour;
◆ religion;

◆ politics;
◆ sexual orientation;
◆ marital status;
◆ hair colour;
◆ type or style of clothing;
◆ height;
◆ weight;
◆ age.

Many job application forms now have two sections, one for career information, the other for personal information. The two sections are separated before going to the short-listing panel so that a decision is based solely on the career section. Despite this, prejudices still surface.

One panel member may dislike writing that slopes to the left and therefore discriminate against that candidate, probably in an unconscious way.

Prejudices are often related to stereotypes and involve what appear to others to be illogical and emotional thoughts and actions but which are quite logical to the individual concerned. The object of the prejudice is different in some way from the 'norm', as perceived by the individual who labels the object. For example, a white Englishman could be non prejudiced against a white Dutchman yet be prejudiced against another Englishman who happens to be black.

Hardy and Heyes (1999) have described an experiment carried out in a primary school by the teacher, Jane Elliot (Box 4.6).

What the experiments described in Box 4.6 demonstrate is how irrational and discriminatory prejudices are. Much of the research into how prejudices can be reduced has shown that if inter-group teams are constructed, with equal status in the group between members, and common goals to work towards, then reductions do occur.

To achieve a reduction in prejudice in the nursing environment is potentially difficult because of the mix of grades. However, if each person in the team is made to feel that they have an equal contribution to make to the running of the ward or unit, then prejudices will be reduced. To be more successful, this concept would need to involve all

---

Box 4.6 Prejudice

A teacher, Jane Elliot, told her class of 9-year-olds that those with brown eyes were more intelligent than those with blue eyes (she had blue eyes herself).

Rules were laid down, such as the 'inferior' students were to sit at the back of the class and use proper cups instead of the drinking fountain. The 'superior' students were given extra privileges. The blue-eyed children although in the majority, became depressed, angry and sullen. They attributed negative words to themselves such as 'dull' and 'stupid'. This became a self-fulfilling prophecy in a remarkably short time (within minutes). The blue-eyed children became nasty and vicious.

The next day, Mrs Elliot stated she had made a mistake, and that it was really the brown-eyed children who were inferior. Almost immediately they reverted to the same behaviour as the blue-eyed children the day before. An interesting point was that many of the brown-eyed children had black skin, but this was disregarded by the white children in the fight against the common enemy.

This same experiment has been repeated in a more sophisticated form with adults, with similar results. The experiment raised a number of ethical questions and for this reason, participants were fully debriefed on each occasion, resulting in a mixture of relief and laughter.

---

members of the multidisciplinary team, including the patient.

In this situation individual prejudices can be submerged in striving for the common goal. However, they could still surface unconsciously in the ways in which a nurse might interact non-verbally with a patient. For example, the patient may be referred to as:

◆ the child-batterer;
◆ the patient with scar tissue of face or hands;
◆ the patient with a different religious viewpoint;
◆ the demanding patient.

It is useful to reflect on prejudices and to devise strategies to reduce them.

PERCEPTUAL DISTORTIONS

In order to pay attention, the perception of a stimulus needs to occur, and yet distortions can happen. Perception is extremely selective. If it were not, there would be a hopeless jumble of sounds, scents, sights and sensations, all competing for attention and causing sensory overload.

In Activity 4.4 although two people might hear the same sounds, each will be selective in their perception of that sound. The chances are that a sound which is heard outside the room illicits the response 'It sounds like…'.

Activity 4.4 Perceptual distortions

Sit in a chair in a familiar room. Have someone else sit in another chair. Both close your eyes for 2 minutes. Concentrate on the sounds within and around you, in the room and outside. When you open your eyes, write down all the things you heard and compare your list with the other person. You will notice many similarities but also some differences.

The brain has to rely on incoming information via the senses to identify what is a stimulus. It is constantly comparing a sound, smell, sight or touch with the 'memory bank' of similar sensations.

If a loud bang is heard outside, the response could be 'that sounds like a car backfiring'. Another person hearing the same sound may say 'that sounds like a gun being fired'. Each person hears the same sound, yet 'perceives' it differently. Without being present to see what caused the sound, each individual makes an assumption based on his past experience of the same or a similar sound and each individual defines what the sound is almost before it is 'heard'.

In Activity 4.5, most people identify three 'F's. Actually there are five. The 'F' in 'of' sounds like a 'v' and so disappears. Perception of the outside world is similar enough for most people to enable them to communicate using common definitions (e.g. red, tree, B. flat). However, it is wrong to assume that what one person 'sees' is always what everyone else 'sees'. The magician's illusion is a classical example.

Activity 4.5 Anticipating stimuli

The anticipation of stimuli is called a perceptual set. In the following sentence count how many times the letter F appears. Forty-four people were of more than average build in the scientific study carried out of teenage school children.

The audience 'see' the assistant disappearing from the box, but another magician will see a false panel knowing how the trick is done. The audience know that the assistant hasn't really disappeared because they have seen the trick performed before. However, the illusion is so strong, that it still causes the brain to perceive an impossible event. The second magician, because of his training, was able to perceive things that the audience did not. Similarly, an experienced nurse, a student nurse and a patient will perceive the same stimuli in different ways, based on their level of understanding, beliefs, values and past experiences. All the factors mentioned in this chapter can contribute to differing interpretations of the same event.

A patient who is having a surgical wound redressed for the first time, may perceive all the equipment as threatening and may anticipate a considerable amount of pain. A student nurse would perceive this situation as an opportunity to practise her newly acquired skills of aseptic technique, and would be concentrating on remembering the sequence of cleansing the wound and manipulating the forceps. An experienced nurse would perceive the situation as an opportunity to converse with the patient, to put him at ease and assess the condition of the wound. The nurse would then determine what action to take in relation to the dressing of the wound, based on her experience of other similar wounds. Each of the three persons has different perceptual sets of the same stimuli.

All these factors show ways in which an individual filters incoming stimuli from the world and creates a unique view of that world. People do interact with each other in different contexts and it is the effects of these contexts which are now discussed.

COMMUNICATION IN CONTEXT

In the previous section, the way in which an individual perceives certain stimuli was discussed. This perception is influenced by the context. For example the symbol 13 can be perceived as the letter B or the number 13 depending upon the context (A B C D or 12 13 14 15).

Describing the context in which communication takes place uses an interactionist approach. It takes into account not only internal factors, but also the role perceptions of the people involved and the external constraints imposed upon the interaction. Baron and Byrne (1994) cite the example of a woman who becomes pregnant. The woman may see this as an 'accident'. The obstetrician who runs a fertility clinic may, on the other hand, see this as successful high fertility on the part of the woman and her husband. The same behaviour is attributed to different causes, depending on who is observing it.

Alternatively, behaviour could be modified according to the context. An office worker would probably communicate differently at a formal dinner party with his boss, than when eating a pub lunch with a group of friends.

Another aspect of context is the way in which people remember certain events. Memories of events are not a random set of mental associations, but a re-creation of the context of that event. This

is known by cognitive psychologists as context-dependent coding, and is best illustrated through hearing a favourite tune.

Memories of where the tune was first heard, what the person was doing, and even emotions associated with it come flooding back.

CULTURE IN CONTEXT

People from differing cultures are coming together more and more as world travel becomes increasingly accessible. It is important therefore to consider the way in which culture influences communication.

In the last 30 years, much research has been carried out into the way in which culture affects communication, particularly in nonverbal communication. For a more comprehensive discussion of this area see Argyle (1990) and Morris (1978).

The complexities of nonverbal communication in different cultures create a potential minefield with respect to common understanding. For example, if a left-handed British person were to hold out his left hand to shake hands when meeting a Moslem, he would greatly insult the Moslem because, in the latter's culture, this is the hand that is used for, and is therefore associated with, cleaning up after excretion.

Public bodily contact between acquaintances, for example embracing and kissing, is not the norm in Britain whereas it is common in French and Latin cultures. Arabs and Latin Americans stand in close proximity to one another when conversing, yet Swedes and Scots are more distant. The gesture for 'OK' in Britain is usually a circle formed by the thumb and index finger, with the other fingers pointing upwards. To a Tunisian this same signal means 'I am going to kill you'. In some cultures respect for another is shown by avoiding direct eye contact, whereas in other cultures, this lack of eye contact would indicate lack of interest, or suggest that the individual was being dishonest.

The use of silence in communication varies between cultures and sometimes within cultures. In the Western world, silence in conversation is viewed in a negative way. It tends to indicate unwillingness to communicate or lack of interest. In Eastern cultures however, silence is frequently used and the expression of thoughts and feelings is discouraged. This can create problems when people from an Eastern culture apply for jobs with a Western company. When asked at interview to discuss thoughts or feelings, or to express themselves, they would have great difficulty. To do so readily would be a sign of insincerity or boasting. Lack of eye contact might lead the interviewer to perceive that they were underconfident.

Emotional expression varies between cultures. For example, a British person who receives a telephone call to say his mother has died may stand up and excuse himself from the meeting he has been attending. An Italian would probably be more demonstrative in the expression of his sudden grief.

Funerals are characterised by differences in expression of emotion. The British reaction to any pain, either physical or emotional, is to remain calm and to keep the emotions under control. However, the Latin approach is to express emotions freely. In some Asian cultures there are women whose function both before and after funerals, is to wail loudly over the body of the deceased. This is both accepted and expected behaviour.

These examples may be overgeneralisations and it is important that nurses should avoid falling into the trap of stereotyping and labelling people from different cultures.

This perception can be generalised to any patient who does not fit into the role of the ideal patient, a person who is quiet, cooperative and undemanding. The effect of the nonstereotypical patient is documented in research carried out by Stockwell (1972). She found that patients were likely to be avoided by nurses if they were non-British, in hospital for more than 3 months, or who regularly questioned their care and did not comply with routines.

Such unpopular patients did not receive individual holistic care. They were labelled nuisances or hypochondriacs. This could even lead to the withholding of medication to control pain. The more popular, uncomplaining patient could receive better pain control than the very expressive patient. When a behaviour is seen in context, misinterpretation about why the behaviour is taking place can be avoided.

IMPLICATIONS FOR PRACTICE

This section will apply the concepts discussed in the chapter to specific client groups. These are:

◆ the child;
◆ the mentally ill;
◆ the person with learning disabilities;
◆ the elderly.

The child

As discussed at the beginning of this chapter, children have a different perspective on the world depending upon their stage of development. Therefore, when working with children in a clinical or community setting, these differences need to be taken into account. It has been recognised for some time that play serves as an important means of expression and learning for children. According to Flanagan (1996) the desire for play is innate and is only found in higher mammals. It is not only found in children of course; adults engage in play in the form of organised games or less formal activities. Play helps children to explore their relationships with other people and objects and to try out new social roles such as 'mummies and daddies' and 'teachers and pupils'.

The cognitive approach to play is that it is a means for the child to problem solve and to copy the more advanced language of an older child.

The psychodynamic perspective would be that play is a cathartic experience which relieves pent-up emotions. Art has been used to help children express their feelings following traumatic events such as abuse or accidents.

The biological perspective is that play is a way of relieving excess energy.

The behaviourist approach is that a child's behaviour can be shaped by the positive or negative responses they elicit from others when carrying out certain behaviours. If a child is given attention by his parents for throwing a tantrum but not when sitting quietly, he is more likely to continue the negative behaviour.

The humanistic perspective is that play is a means of developing social awareness, empathy with others and acting out emotions.

In clinical settings provision for play has been introduced over the last 30 years, with the purchase of equipment and the employing of nursery nurses. Procedures which children are about to undergo have been integrated into role play using dolls or teddies to play them, their parents and the health care professionals involved.

Lindon (1998) points out that children don't learn just from play. They learn a lot about more abstract concepts from discussions with adults and this can take time and patience. Because staff tend to see play as the only time for children to learn, they don't spend time listening to children's questions as perhaps a parent would at home, so opportunities are missed to check out the child's perception of what is happening to them. It is therefore useful to have a policy of parents staying in hospital with their child.

Curry and Arnaud (1984) suggest that parents and other adults should join in with the child who is playing and talk out loud the thoughts/ideas which are being expressed as well as suggesting elaborations to the game.

The mentally ill

A person who is suffering from a mental illness has a distorted perception of reality which is manifested in different ways depending upon the nature of the illness, the stage of treatment and the individual's psychological makeup. This can vary between acute anxiety states through to psychosis.

One of the causes of acute anxiety is a pathological fear of an object, living animal or situation which, to others, seems irrational – known as a phobia. There are at least 200 known phobias including the more common ones such as: claustraphobia (a fear of confined spaces); arachnophobia (a fear of spiders); and xenophobia (a fear of other races).

Other, less common phobias include fear of mirrors, bananas, all animals and even fear of fear itself (panphobia). Although the person suffering from the phobia may be aware that the fear is irrational, they are unable to prevent the anxiety state from arising. Phobias can be overcome by desensitisation whereby the individual is exposed to the least-threatening aspect of the stimulus such as a photograph of a spider. If the person is able to tolerate this, they will then go on to be shown a dead spider, then, successively, a live spider in a glass cage, then one running free on a table and, if the person is able to tolerate it, to have the spider run over their hand. If at any point, the person exhibits signs or symptoms of increasing anxiety, the therapist will move them back one stage until they feel comfortable. This is a form of behavioural therapy where there is a reward linked to acceptable behaviour.

Similar techniques have been used in psychiatric institutions whereby patients who exhibit socially accepted behaviours were 'rewarded' with tokens which could be exchanged for goods at the hospital shop. Socially unacceptable behaviours were ignored. This led to a gradual extinction of the unacceptable behaviours. This same approach has been used with patients who have a learning disability.

In psychosis, the individual's thought processes are affected in that they may be experiencing hallucinations such as sights, sounds and smells which to the observer are not there. Or they may be suffering from delusions which are beliefs or ideas with no basis in reality. Often, an initial false belief can lead to the development of a web of quite logical thoughts, ideas and behaviours. For example, the person may believe that they have vast amounts of wealth and therefore feel free to telephone hire firms, and staff at the hospital then have the embarrassing prospect of 10 stretch limousines turning up at the hospital.

It is difficult trying to convince someone that what they are experiencing is not real. This requires specialist knowledge and communication strategies outside the scope of this book.

The person with learning disabilities

The term 'learning disability' has only been in use in the UK in the last 15 years. Prior to that, terms such as 'mentally handicapped' and 'mentally defective' were used. Historically, people with a learning disability were seen as second-class citizens and were cared for in large institutional settings away from mainstream society, often alongside patients with a mental illness. There are many examples of men and women with mild forms of learning disability who were in locked institutions for most of their lives. Following a document known as *Better Services for The Mentally Handicapped* (DHSS 1971), the emphasis gradually moved from institutional care to the setting up of services in the community under local authority control. This led to the setting up of small, staffed homes within community settings. There were many objections to this from local residents as perceptions of those with a learning disability were that they would be noisy, violent and promiscuous. This is a good example of misplaced assumptions, stereotyping and prejudicial attitudes which were sometimes fuelled by sensational tabloid newspaper headlines.

As discussed earlier in this chapter attitudes, beliefs and values are often difficult to change and, in the case of learning disability, this process has taken several years. With this in mind, it is vital that health care professionals act in a way which is nonjudgemental, accepting and warm. Carl Rogers (1980) described this as 'unconditional positive regard'. Along with this, the practitioner needs to be aware of the comprehension level of the client when communicating information.

There is a tendency for many people with a learning disability to be unaware of the social norms in relation to nonverbal communication, especially spatial awareness and touch. The practitioner may therefore have to set the boundaries for this and make sure that they also apply the same boundaries to themselves so that they don't come across as being patronising.

For a comprehensive review of learning disability practice read Gates and Beacock (1997).

The elderly

As a person grows older the effects of the ageing process become evident. The five senses diminish, skin and connective tissue lose their elasticity and organs including the brain begin to function less efficiently. This can happen at different rates in different people. There are some very fit, alert 80-year-olds and some very frail, confused 60-year-olds. It is important therefore that nurses don't stereotype or label someone who is over a certain age as hard of hearing or demented.

Unfortunately, because of this tendency to perceive the elderly person as less than proficient physically or mentally, a certain amount of stereotyping can occur. For example, language is modified when talking to an elderly person. There is a tendency to use 'baby talk' which sends the message to the older person, 'You are less capable than you once were, and I have less affection for you than I once did.' Unfortunately, this is reinforced because there is a slight increase in reaction time when someone is hard of hearing which is perceived as evidence of diminished cognitive capacity. Also, if the elderly individual feels as though they are being treated as a simpleton or as a child this may increase anxiety.

In reality only about 15% of people aged over 75 years are hard of hearing, with another 20% suffering from hearing impairment (Darbyshire 1984). Speech should be slower but not louder because facial expressions change when the voice is raised and the tone goes higher. When a person is becoming hard of hearing, the perception of higher tones go first so this is counterproductive. Also, there is a tendency to move closer when speaking to someone who is hard of hearing. This involves invading the body space of the other person and can be inhibiting or threatening. The person is also unable to lip read and thus loses parts of the message.

Another problem when communicating with the elderly is that carers often invalidate statements made by them. For example, if a person states 'I don't feel well' and the other person responds 'Oh, that's too bad' then validation has occurred. If, on the other hand, the other person either does not respond or states 'Oh yes you do – you feel just fine' than the first statement has been invalidated. Another form of invalidation is if one person states 'I don't feel well' and the other person states 'I'm feeling pretty good today.'. These sorts of responses can make the other person doubt their sense of self and self-concept. If this happens often enough, the elderly person can have their self-esteem weakened. Unfortunately, this does happen in many continuing care settings. This invalidation of a person can of course work the other way in that an elderly person may forget what a carer has said to them or could even forget who the carer is. This then invalidates the younger person. A combination of these factors could lead to a very unfulfilling relationship between the elderly person and their carer.

Another misconception about the elderly is that there is a decline in intellectual functioning. Niven (2000) cites several longitudinal research studies which indicate that, in the absence of organic brain disease, if a person has been intellectually active during adulthood they will continue to be so in old age. There is a slowing down in reaction time and sometimes problems with encoding and retrieval of memory. Therefore, health professionals should allow time for the elderly person to make decisions and should provide 'aides-memoire' to help with memory recall. In long-term institutions the residents could be involved in organising their day-to-day activities along with special events.

CONCLUSION

Communication is a complex process involving both interpersonal and intrapersonal factors. Each person is a unique individual, with a unique interpretation of the world, influenced by origin, upbringing and life experience.

What seems certain is the lack of simple conclusive answers to describe the uniqueness of the individual, although some factors, particularly internal ones, can be described, for example, defence mechanisms, attitudes, assumptions, prejudices and perceptual distortions.

These factors modify external stimuli and determine the way in which a person will respond to them. The physical and cultural contexts of the interaction are also important.

Nurses need to be aware of these factors and be able to see them in themselves as well as in their patients/clients. This will help them to empathise and interact in a meaningful way with others. This chapter has also explored differences between the range of client groups that nurses encounter during their practice. There have necessarily been some generalisations made about these groups and there will be individual differences between clients. The reader is advised to consult more detailed texts in those areas.

The debate about nature versus nurture has been put back firmly on the agenda as a result of recent discoveries about the function of genes and the ability to 'map' them. The spectre of eugenics and issues of cloning have come into the debate as a result of these discoveries. Because of the complexities of human beings and their experiences, it would seem that there is a mix of nature and nurture involved. As Jawaharal Nehru once said, 'Life is like a game of cards. The hand that is dealt you represents determinism. The way you play it is free will'.

In the following example taken from an authentic situation it is possible to identify some of the areas that have been discussed in this chapter. The skill is to determine ways in which the outcome described here could have been avoided (Box 4.7).

Communication is about being aware of the way in which messages can be influenced by all the factors discussed. A way of checking one's own perception is by the use of meta-communication and feedback. By doing this, other people in the interaction will perceive that they are relating to someone, who, as Carl Rogers (1980) would say, is showing unconditional positive regard and empathetic understanding.

Box 4.7 Miscommunication

Staff Nurse Murphy was arriving on the night shift in the operating theatre. She was told by the departing staff nurse that the theatre needed preparing for Dr. Ahmed, who was operating on Abraham Liddle first thing in the morning. When the staff nurse left, Nurse Murphy realised that she had not been told what operation the patient was having. She rang round the wards to find out about Abraham Liddle. All the wards she contacted had no patient by that name. By now the time was 12 midnight. Staff Nurse Murphy decided to call the surgeon. Dr. Ahmed had been asleep for 1 hour when the telephone rang.

He was upset at being woken over such a trivial matter, and at such a late hour, when he needed to sleep. He answered the nurse sharply, stating that of course the patient existed, he had examined him that afternoon and he did not want to be disturbed again. He then banged the phone down. The Staff Nurse, upset and angry at the doctor's response to a perfectly reasonable request, attempted to locate the patient again, without success. She prepared the theatre for general surgery as best she could.

The next night she returned to duty to be confronted by an irate theatre sister, who stated that the theatre list had been held for an hour that morning, because the Abraham Needle which Dr. Ahmed had needed to carry out a liver biopsy on his first patient, Mr. Johnstone, was not available as had been requested.

REFERENCES

Adler RB, Rodman G 1991 Understanding human communication, 4th edn. Holt, Rinehart, Winston, Florida

Argyle M 1990 Bodily communication, 2nd edn. Routledge, London

Baron RA, Byrne D 1994 Social psychology – understanding human interactions, 7th edn. Allyn & Bacon, Boston, USA

Bremmer A, Bryant P 2001 The effect of spatial cues on infant responses in the AB task, with and without a hidden object. Developmental Science 4(4): 408–415

Couzigou P, Begleiter H, Kiianmaa K 1999 Alcohol and genetics. In: MacDonald I (ed) Health issues related to alcohol consumption. Blackwell Science, Oxford

Curry NE, Arnaud S 1984 Play in pre-school settings. In: Yawkey T, Pellegrini A (eds) Child's play, developmental & applied. Lawrence Erlbaum, London

Darbyshire J 1984 The hearing loss epidemic: A challenge to gerontology. Research on Aging 6: 384–394

Department of Health and Social Security 1971 Better services for the mentally handicapped. HMSO, London

Emslie GR 1979 The psychoanalytical approach. In: Medcof J, Roth J (eds) Approaches to psychology. Open University Press, Milton Keynes

Festinger L 1957 A theory of cognitive dissonance. Paterson, Evanston Row

Flanagan C 1996 Applying psychology to early child development. Hodder & Stoughton, London

Freud A 1946 The ego and mechanisms of defence. Karnac Books, London

Freud S 1954 The origins of psychoanalysis. Basic Books, New York

Gates B, Beacock C 1997 Dimensions of learning disability. Baillière Tindall, London

Glover D 1985 The sociology of the mass media. In: Haralambos M (ed) Sociology new directions. Causeway Press, Ormskirk

Hargie O (ed) 1997 The handbook of communication skills, 2nd edn. Routledge, London

Hardy M, Heyes S 1999 Beginning psychology, 5th edn. Oxford University Press, Oxford

Heider F 1958 The psychology of interpersonal relations. Wiley, New York

Jaroff L 1989 The Gene Hunt. Time Magazine 20th March, pp. 62–67

Kagan C, Evans J, Kay B 1986 A manual of interpersonal skills for nurses – an experiential approach. Harper & Row, London

Lindon J 1998 Understanding child development. MacMillan Press, Basingstoke

Maslow A 1954 Motivation and personality. Harper & Row, New York

Morris D 1978 Manwatching: a field guide to human behaviour. Cape, London

Niven N 2000 Health psychology for health care professionals, 3rd edn. Churchill Livingstone, Edinburgh

Oxford English Dictionary 1998 University Press, Oxford

Peele S 1990 Second thoughts about a gene for alcoholism. The Atlantic Monthly August: 52–58

Piaget J, Inhelder B 1969 The psychology of the child. Routledge & Kegan Paul, London

Pluckman ML 1978 Human communication: the matrix of nursing. McGraw Hill, New York

Rogers CR 1980 A way of being. Houghton Mifflin, Boston

Sinsheimer RL 1991 The human genome initiative. FASEB Journal 5: 2885

Stockwell F 1972 The unpopular patient. Royal College of Nursing, London

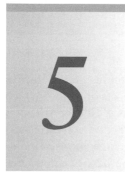

Improving communication

Andy Betts

5

INTRODUCTION

When two people engage in conversation much more is taking place than the observer sees. Each person brings his own unique world and perceptions to the encounter in which a multifaceted and apparently infinite collection of stimuli and data are involved. It is hard to imagine how people could proceed through everyday life if they were to pay attention to every minute detail of communication. The human brain instantaneously and efficiently filters the thousands of cues and messages thus preventing the overloading of data. This filtering process is not predominantly a conscious activity. This chapter identifies those factors that cause problems in communication and focuses on what may be done to improve the effectiveness of communication in nursing.

COMMUNICATION AND HEALTH CARE

Studies over the last three decades identify communication problems as persistent causes for concern in the delivery of health care (Menzies 1970, Stockwell 1972, Hayward 1975, Macleod-Clark 1984, Faulkner 1985, Ley 1988, Bradley & Edinberg 1990, Burnard & Morrison 1991, Davis & Fallowfield 1991, Wilkinson 1992, Hewison 1995). Some work in the UK has suggested a direct correlation between communication and patient overall satisfaction (Pagano & Ragan 1992, Meryn 1998). Nursing curricula have been modified in response to these findings but there remains little room for complacency. Indeed there is some evidence to suggest that the latest pre-registration curriculum changes in the UK have resulted in a fragmented, nonexplicit delivery of communication and interpersonal skills (Chant et al 2002).

The reasons for the problems are complex and often specific to the area being researched. Those commonly cited include: lack of skills and training, lack of resources and time, emotional vulnerability, the location of power, and some deliberately perpetuated bad practices between agencies. Perhaps this is no different to the picture in other fields of human encounter when one considers the complexities of communication. Also, the context in which nursing takes place is an elaborate network of relationships with patients, colleagues, informal carers and allied agencies. The potential for things to go wrong is considerable.

Peplau (1988) suggests that nursing is essentially an interpersonal process. If this is the case, then competent nurses are required to be effective communicators and all nurse have a responsibility to pay adequate attention to their own development in this domain. This chapter is grounded in the belief that individuals can become more effective communicators. The pursuit of perfection in communication is a frustrating process. Frustrating because it is lifelong and everyday experiences serve to remind us just how complex and elusive effective communication actually is. Frustrating because to become more effective requires a realisation of inadequacies.

The nature of the problem

There are four major factors that contribute to communication problems in nursing:

- ◆ lack of self-awareness;
- ◆ lack of systematic interpersonal skills training;
- ◆ lack of a conceptual framework;
- ◆ lack of clarity of purpose.

These factors will each be examined in turn.

Lack of self-awareness

One reason why communication may be ineffective is the lack of awareness of aspects of oneself which significantly affect interactions with others. Facets of the individual which are beyond consciousness are also beyond control and become 'loose cannons' which may blow a hole in the best of intentions. The personal factors which affect communication are attitudes, values, beliefs, feelings and behaviours. Increasing self-awareness in these domains is likely to result in more productive interactions and a more intentional use of self. This increased self-understanding serves to convert potential pitfalls into potential assets (Box 5.1).

The realisation that the image one has of oneself may contrast significantly with how one is perceived by others is significant learning and lies at the heart of developing as a communicator. Individuals acquire a subjective view of the world which is different to how others perceive it and much of behaviour is partly unconsciously motivated.

Box 5.1 Increasing self-awareness

Julie, a student on the learning disabilities branch, watches the replay of a video recording of herself interacting with a fellow student. She is both fascinated and disconcerted by what she observes. Seeing herself from the outside presents a contrasting image to the 'internal' view she has of herself.

She notices repeated mannerisms which previously she had no idea she used. She is able to check out later with her peers how they had experienced these behaviours and is not too surprised to discover that they had been perceived as a distraction by others. As a result of this experience Julie is aware of aspects of herself which were previously beyond her consciousness. This learning experience has increased her options and further refined her capacity to communicate effectively with others.

Both of these observations mean that nurses, who are directly involved in interpersonal relationships, need to maximise their self-awareness and conscious use of self. Stein-Parbury (1993) states:

> Nurses need to develop acute self-awareness whenever they engage in interactions and relationships with patients, because the primary tool they are using in these circumstances is themselves. Without self-awareness nurses run the risk of imposing their values and views onto patients. Through self-awareness nurses remain in touch with what they are doing and how this is affecting patients for whom they care.
> (Stein-Parbury, p. 60)

One important characteristic of human communication is that not all signals and messages are sent intentionally or even consciously (see Chapter 1). There is often a discrepancy between what the individual perceives during communication and other people's understanding. This has important implications for the nurse as a communicator because it is this potential discrepancy which leads to all kinds of problems in communication. Effective communication requires people to maximise self-awareness, both in terms of how behaviour is perceived by others and also in understanding one's own motivations and blind spots.

Lack of systematic interpersonal skills training

The use of the words 'systematic' and 'training' is highly significant and controversial in the context of interpersonal skills. To some degree communication consists of a set of skills. These are the 'tools of the trade of communication'. As such, the most effective method of becoming competent in using them is the same as for any skills training. Of course, communication is much more than a technology but systematic skills training has a role to play in becoming an effective communicator.

There is a reluctance to accept this not that communication will, in some way, be reduced to a dehumanised series of mechanistic behaviours and formulae. This does not apply to other aspects of the nurse's role such as carrying out complex clinical procedures. In these cases the skills are practised until competence is achieved.

Systematic interpersonal skills training, if structured correctly, does not result in homogenised cloning but competent communicators who have integrated identified skills into their unique style of communication. The systematic training in the use of microskills is just the first step in a process that must lead to these skills becoming second nature (Patterson 1988).

Chapter 2 includes some description of human development and a clue as to why things may go wrong is revealed by examining how people learn to communicate. An important part of a child's development is to learn to communicate effectively but, surprisingly, this is left largely to chance. It is acquired mainly from parents, the significant role models in early life, and also from other influential grown ups and peers. It would appear that this learning process works amazingly well. The capabilities of even a preschool child to communicate using a wide-ranging vocabulary are impressive. By the age of physical maturity most are capable of a complex repertoire of interactions.

On a different level, however, it is possible to be critical of the absence of systematic interpersonal skills training. If, as seems to be the case, children acquire skills as they go along it would appear that they are also likely to learn some of the 'bad habits' of their role models and lack the awareness necessary to discriminate between what is effective and what is not. The consequences for nursing are significant. Egan (1998) notes that those entering the helping professions often do not possess the basic set of helping skills. Historically, nursing curricula have failed to address this deficit although there has been an increasing emphasis on interpersonal skills training in recent years with varying degrees of success (Dunn 1991).

Lack of a conceptual framework

Nurses who demonstrate competence in the application of interpersonal skills may sometimes use them in an ad hoc fashion (Dunn 1991). A theoretical framework is required which informs communication and provides a structure for the analysis, reflection and evaluation of interactions. Given the complexities highlighted in previous chapters, attempting to understand communication without a framework is problematic. It is important for nurses to be able to conceptualise what they are doing to ensure that skills are used in a coherent and strategic manner. Such a framework provides the language and conceptual organisation to make sense of interactions both retrospectively and as they occur. Although many different theories and models exist to explain different aspects of the nurse's role, e.g. nursing care models, counselling models, management models and supervision models, there are far fewer theories designed to focus solely on communication. Two such theories will be considered later in this chapter.

Lack of clarity of purpose

On a conscious level communication is concerned with making choices. The effective communicator has a high success rate of making appropriate choices for the situations that are encountered because he is clear about the aims or purpose of each interaction (Heron 1990). This enables the effective communicator to discriminate between alternative choices, selecting what suits a specific situation. It is not usually the nurse who determines the purpose of the interaction but the needs of the client. This process requires sensitivity and empathy (see Chapter 7) to enable the nurse to read the situation accurately and assess what is required. For example, the communication skills required in giving advice on a specific subject are significantly different to those required to listen to a distressed individual. Developing the ability to read situations, to be clear about the intention and to pursue it strategically are the hallmarks of effective communication.

IMPROVING COMMUNICATION BY ADDRESSING DEFICITS

Increasing self-awareness

Burnard (1985) defines self-awareness as a process. He observes that:

> Self-awareness refers to the gradual and continuous process of noticing and exploring aspects of self, whether behavioural, psychological or physical, with the intention of developing personal and interpersonal understanding to have a deeper understanding of ourselves is to have a sharper and clearer picture of what is happening to others.
> In a sense it is a process of discrimination.
> (Burnard, 1985, pp. 15–16)

This concept of discrimination is linked to ideas discussed in Chapter 1, in the context of internal and external worlds. Recognising differences and similarities to others is an important aspect of work in human care services.

Rogers (1967) emphasised that understanding oneself is a significant prerequisite to understanding others but to what extent this is achievable is open to question. The idea that self-awareness can be achieved on a certain day may sound ridiculous. The concept of self-awareness is best thought of as a continuum. The lifelong task is to inch along that continuum in the realisation and acceptance that the end may never be reached. Any progress made is through introspective processes such as reflection, self-exploration and self-assessment and by interactive activities such as self-disclosure, discussion and feedback. In addition, some may choose to enter a counselling or psychotherapeutic relationship in a deliberate attempt to heighten self-awareness (see Chapter 7).

Learning through reflection

The term 'reflective practitioner' has appeared consistently in the nursing literature since Schon

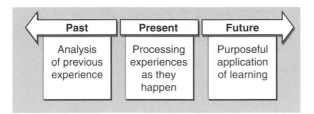

Fig 5.1 Three dimensions of reflection

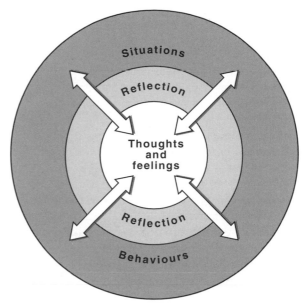

Fig 5.2 Internal and external aspects of reflection

(1983) defined the concept. Nurses seek to incorporate reflection into their practice but confusion exists regarding the meaning of the word. Boud et al (1985) state succinctly that reflection in this context refers to 'turning experience into learning'. This is a purposeful and conscious activity requiring structured time and effort rather than an automatic process. Different methods can be used to achieve this, such as introspection, writing or discussion. One common misconception of reflection is that it consists purely of historical analysis (see Fig. 5.1). Kemmis (1985) stresses that reflection is not an end in itself but that it leads to informed, committed action. Development as a reflective communicator eventually leads to the ability to process what is happening during an interaction rather than after it has finished. Accurate processing of communication as it occurs increases options and results in a more intentional use of self.

Reflection involves both inward and outward activities (see Fig. 5.2). The inward activity is concerned with paying attention to thoughts and feelings and the external focus is on the situation and behaviours. Asking questions, hypothesising, reality testing and evaluating are all activities closely linked to the concept of reflection. It is productive to 'replay' interactions in which we were involved. To picture oneself back in the situation and process what happened in some detail. For some people reflective writing is productive as a medium for the recording and analysis of interactions. The use of learning journals or communication diaries to record analytic and evaluative introspection are structures which may suit some people. Walker (1985) suggests that writing provides an objectivity

and clarity to experiences by removing elements of subjective feeling that can obscure issues. These written records also provide data for further review in tutorials, supervision sessions or with peers. Some examples of reflective questions are given in Box 5.2.

Learning from feedback

Dickson et al (1989) discriminate between two types of feedback in relation to communication skills. Intrinsic feedback is an integral feature of any interaction. Information is available from others involved during an interaction which indicates their responses to specific interventions. Learning to pay attention to intrinsic feedback during interactions and then responding accordingly is an important component of effective communication. Learning to concentrate sensitively on the cues and responses of the people with whom you are communicating helps in understanding the process of communication and informs the choice of response made. Extrinsic feedback refers to explicit

Box 5.2 Examples of reflective questions

What was the context of the interaction?
What actually happened?
What was my reaction to what happened?
What were my behaviours, thoughts, feelings at the time?
What was the behaviour of the other(s)?
What do I imagine were the other'(s) thoughts and feelings at the time?
What were my thoughts and feelings afterwards?
What do I imagine were the other'(s) thoughts and feelings afterwards?
What was the purpose of the interaction?
How successful was the interaction?
What skills did I use well/not so well?
Given the opportunity how would I do it differently?

Box 5.3 Principles of giving and receiving feedback

Giving feedback
1. Be specific. A clear statement of what precisely was observed is more helpful than a wide generalisation.

2. Achieve a balance. Highlight the strengths but also include aspects which require attention. Praise alone may make the person feel good but is not as helpful as balanced feedback.

3. Offer possible alternatives. Comment tentatively on how things could have been done differently. Avoid dogmatic advice.

4. Refer to behaviour rather than personal characteristics. Behaviour can be changed; personal characteristics cannot.

5. If a contract exists, stay within its boundaries, i.e. if specific feedback is requested then this should be the focus of your comments.

6. Think what your feedback says about you.

Receiving feedback
1. Have an open mind. Avoid becoming defensive or argumentative and do not reject the feedback.

2. Ask for clarification.

3. Listen, consider and decide what you will do in the light of the feedback.

information provided by others directly relating to the interactions. For example, a student on a placement contract might accompany his or her mentor and focus particularly on his listening skills to observe and comment on an interaction with a client. The feedback in this case is supplementary to the actual interaction.

Both types of feedback are fundamental elements to improving communication skills. In the absence of extrinsic feedback the only perspective available is a subjective view which includes blind spots and limiting perceptions. Feedback serves the following functions:

◆ Promotion of self-awareness through the assimilation of information about how one is seen by others.
◆ Increase of options. More information provides new perspectives and different choices.
◆ Reinforcement. Positive feedback is likely to increase the frequency of productive behaviour.
◆ Encouragement and motivation. A working culture which incorporates constructive feedback tends to result in employees feeling more valued.

Providing feedback to others is in itself a communication skill and as such may be delivered constructively or destructively. Constructive feedback results in the four outcomes stated above. Destructive feedback leaves the recipient feeling negative and unclear about how to improve matters. Learning to provide constructive feedback adds value to the learning process but also has application in most other human interactions. The principles shown in Box 5.3 apply to the giving and receiving of constructive, extrinsic feedback.

Interpersonal skills training

Learning any skill requires progression through a number of different stages from identifying an individual skill through to the eventual mastery and integration of that skill. These stages are described by Egan (1985) and Dickson et al (1989). The following stages represent a training process which is an amalgamation of both descriptions.

Identification of individual nonverbal and verbal microskills appropriate to the context of the communication This stage results in clarity of understanding of what the skills are in terms of definitions, behaviours, aims and application. It is achieved, for example, through reading, lectures and discussions.

Knowledge of how to use the skills This is achieved by observing demonstrations of others using the skills. This may take the form of a live demonstration, video or audio tapes. This stage facilitates progression from conceptual understanding to behavioural understanding.

Practice of the skills The opportunity to try using the skills with peers in structured training sessions either using role play or preferably 'live' issues.

Evaluation of the practice through focused feedback This stage enables reflection on one's own performance and also constructive feedback from peers and teachers. The intention is to confirm what is done well and to correct what is not. A common structure is for a peer to observe the interaction and notice specifically what takes place.

Evaluation of the training process Periodic evaluation of one's overall progress and the experience of the training process is useful in consolidating different experiences.

Implementation in the 'real world' Putting the skills together within a nursing context is the final stage. Moving from the formalised learning environment to the practice setting and gradually integrating what has been learned so that it becomes second nature. This process is made easier by effective supervision, introspective reflection and feedback mechanisms.

A common experience of this learning process is to feel deskilled at different stages. Often nurses feel discouraged by this temporary sense of incompetence.

The hypothetical dialogue in Box 5.4 is between a teacher and a student nurse who is currently studying for a communication and interpersonal skills module. It illustrates some of the potential difficulties.

The learning curve represents a journey. At the beginning of the journey in Box 5.4 the nurse is communicating without thinking too deeply about it. The next step involves thinking about how he communicates but also feeling deskilled. This is followed by a growing sense of competence which still requires much concentration. Finally, the nurse is able to communicate more competently without having to think so consciously about what he is doing.

A knowledge of pragmatic theories

Knowledge of a pragmatic theory of communication enables nurses to conceptualise what they are doing and provides a means to discuss interactions.

Two such theories which serve the purpose well are transactional analysis (Berne 1966) and six category intervention analysis (Heron 1990). The rationale for selecting these examples is that they are exhaustive in the sense that they may be applied to all interpersonal interactions in which nurses are likely to be involved during the course of their work.

Transactional analysis

Transactional analysis (TA) is much more than a framework for the analysis of interactions. It is also a theory of personality and a psychotherapeutic approach. The strengths of the theory lie in robust but simple concepts and their wide application to human encounters. A comprehensive description of the theory is beyond the scope of this text but students are advised to read from the reference section at the end of this chapter for further information.

Box 5.4 The potential difficulties of interpersonal skills training

Student: 'I don't see the purpose of all this time we spend on learning communication skills. I can already communicate. I do it everyday with people. Surely there are more worthwhile subjects on which we could spend this time.'

Teacher: 'I appreciate that you already communicate at a sophisticated level and I hope that the work you are doing here is an acknowledgement of that. The emphasis that is placed on communication in the curriculum is based on the belief that nursing is essentially an interpersonal process and that we can all become more effective than we are right now. What do you think?'

Student: 'I think that we pick up communication as we go through life. If I have to stop to think about everything that I do and say I will be unable to do anything.'

Teacher: 'Unfortunately there is some truth in that. Learning interpersonal skills is difficult precisely because we have to focus on the complex details that we normally do not think about. Paradoxically this can make us feel less effective than when we just get on with it.'

Student: 'So what's the point?'

Teacher: 'The point is that this feeling of being deskilled is only a temporary step on the learning curve. To use an analogy; when you drive your car you are performing extremely complex behaviours, judgements and reactions. The surprising fact is that you are rarely consciously thinking about how you will change gear, steer, use the accelerator and brakes, etc. Somehow you just do it! If you have a passenger with you it is even possible to hold a conversation at the same time as carrying out these functions. Let's say that one day you decide to take advanced driving lessons. Your instructor prompts you to notice aspects of your driving performance by bringing them to your attention. This feels strange almost to the point that you feel you are unable to drive the car at all. Somehow the process has become laboured and disjointed just like it was when you first learned to drive. The feedback from the instructor leads you to do things differently and gradually the activity of driving becomes a different experience again. You become more aware of your strengths as a driver and of the areas you have to work at. Over time you become less clumsy and realise that you have refined skills and corrected bad practices of which you were previously not even aware. Eventually the whole process becomes a smooth concerted performance again but you now know that you are a better driver.'

Student: 'So what you are saying is that we will probably get worse before we get better at communication.'

Teacher: 'This is likely to be how you will experience this part of the course. Being asked to think more deeply about how you communicate is an unusual request but is necessary if you are to ultimately improve your communication with others.'

The main concept of transactional analysis is the ego state. At any one time people manifest a part of their personality in a consistent pattern of behaviour, thoughts and feelings. These distinct patterns are known as ego states.

The three main ego states are indicated in Figure 5.3. The parent ego state refers to when a person behaves, thinks and feels in ways which are copied from his own parents or parental figures. The child ego state refers to a pattern of behaviour, thoughts and feelings which are replayed from one's childhood. The adult ego state refers to behaviours, thoughts and feelings which are direct and appropriate responses to the here and now. None of the ego states have anything to do with time or whether one actually is a parent, adult or child. Young children at play often behave and relate to each other as if one were the parent and the other a child. Similarly, adults sometimes behave as children. Stewart and Joines (1987) suggest that a healthy and balanced personality requires all three of these ego states: 'adult' to enable problem

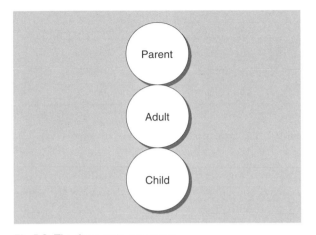

Fig 5.3 The three main ego states

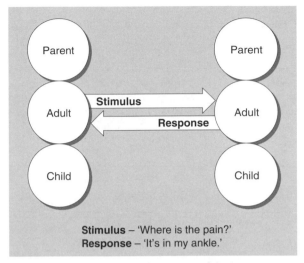

Stimulus – 'Where is the pain?'
Response – 'It's in my ankle.'

Fig 5.4 Adult-to-adult complementary transaction

solving, 'parent' to cope with society and its rules, 'child' for access to spontaneity, creativity and intuition. At any time one of the three ego states usually predominates.

This model provides a useful framework for understanding human interactions. Whenever two people are communicating with each other they are doing so from one of the three ego states. To observe and listen to them it is possible to discriminate between the different ego states and to note shifts that occur. Conceptually there is a way of analysing interactions. A transaction involves a stimulus and a response.

An example of an adult-to-adult complementary transaction is shown in Figure 5.4. The stimulus is a fact-finding question which invites a response from the adult ego state, which answers the question. Complementary transactions refer to those exchanges in which the arrows are parallel and in which the ego state that is addressed is the one that responds. A second example of a complementary transaction involving different ego states is seen in Figure 5.5. The arrows remain parallel.

When transactions are complementary conversation tends to flow back and forth in a consistent manner. If, however, the arrows are crossed rather than parallel in a transaction then there is usually an interruption in communication while individuals shift ego states (see Fig. 5.6).

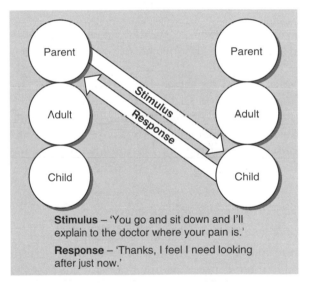

Stimulus – 'You go and sit down and I'll explain to the doctor where your pain is.'

Response – 'Thanks, I feel I need looking after just now.'

Fig 5.5 Parent-to-child complementary transaction

The example of a crossed transaction shows what happens when the ego state which is addressed is not the one which responds. There is usually a feeling of surprise when this happens. The response invites the other person to move into the child ego state, perhaps feeling put down and hurt. An understanding of this analytical framework provides the language and concepts to make sense of

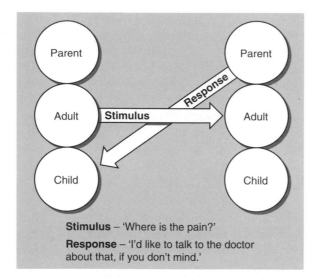

Stimulus – 'Where is the pain?'

Response – 'I'd like to talk to the doctor about that, if you don't mind.'

Fig 5.6 Adult-to-adult, parent-to-child crossed transaction

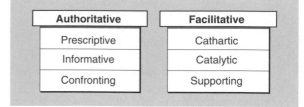

Fig 5.7 Six category intervention analysis (Heron 1990)

Authoritative	Facilitative
Prescriptive	Cathartic
Informative	Catalytic
Confronting	Supporting

everyday interactions. Without such a framework communication is often difficult to process in a coherent manner. Also, the ego state model provides choices for the communicator. Where a language exists to describe what is happening there is more likelihood of seeing alternatives that are available during interactions. In this sense the model provides a structure for retrospective analysis and for informing future goal-directed communication.

Six category intervention analysis

Heron (1990, p. 7) claims six category intervention analysis to be 'exhaustive of the major sorts of valid interventions any practitioner needs to make in relation to clients'.

For nurses, this provides a very useful framework in which to examine their interactions with other people. Just as with transactional analysis, this model offers a conceptual structure to both assist the processing and to inform the choices in nursing communication. The rationale for the inclusion of two such theories is to make the point that each is valid. There is no single complete and authoritative approach to examining such a complex activity as communication. Neither theory is

'real' but together they do provide alternative conceptual binoculars through which to view the world of communication.

Heron has identified six independent categories to classify the different types of interventions. He describes an intervention as 'any identifiable piece of verbal and/or non-verbal behaviour that is part of the practitioner's service to the client' (Heron 1990, p. 3). The categories are shown in Figure 5.7 and are briefly described below.

The authoritative interventions are more directive categories in the sense that the nurse takes responsibility for the client. The facilitative categories are concerned with enabling clients to take responsibility for themselves. It is the context which determines the appropriate category to use. Heron (1990) regards each of the categories as equally valid as long as they are matched to the nurse's role, the client's needs and the purpose of the intervention. Each category includes specific skills and strategies which in turn require competent delivery:

◆ Prescriptive interventions include communication which aims to direct the other's behaviour, such as delegating tasks to colleagues or advising a client about taking medication.

◆ Informative interventions refer to interactions intended to give information, knowledge or meaning. Information is different to advice in that it tends to be more neutral and factual and less socially influencing, for example, explaining about a particular clinical procedure.

◆ Confronting interventions serve the purpose of challenging limiting perspectives, attitudes or behaviours, such as pointing out in a sensitive manner a client's self-defeating pattern of behaviour.

Box 5.5 Six category intervention analysis at work

David is an experienced nurse who works on a children's ward. As he goes about his work he is approached by many different people during a shift. His experience, skills and education help him to choose appropriately how to respond to each encounter. If you were to observe him using six category intervention analysis you would notice how he advises parents about providing care at home; gives information to children in a way that they can understand; confronts a particularly boisterous youngster about his behaviour which is upsetting other children; encourages parents to express their fears about an operation; prompts a child to describe his situation during an assessment; and takes time to show his appreciation to his colleagues for their hard work. What makes David effective in his role is his ability to match skilled responses to the respective situations.

◆ Cathartic interventions enable others to express their emotions. Encouraging bereaved relatives to express the feelings associated with their loss is a case in point.

◆ Catalytic interventions help to draw out information and promote self-discovery and understanding.

◆ Supportive interventions affirm the worth of others and demonstrate respect and acceptance. Using counselling skills or running a support group are examples of this.

The strength of this framework is that it prompts nurses to be clear about the purpose of any communication in which they are involved. One way of thinking about the interventions is to compare them to selecting the most strategic card from a hand of playing cards (see Box 5.5).

The skilled communicator is proficient in all six of the categories and able to move from one to another as the situation requires. Burnard & Morrison (1991) conducted a number of studies looking at nurses' self-evaluation of skills using six category intervention analysis. The findings consistently suggest that nurses evaluate themselves as more skilled in the prescriptive, informative and supportive categories and less skilled in the cathartic, catalytic and confronting categories. A number of possible reasons are suggested for this by the researchers but it may well be that these categories require more attention than they currently receive in nursing curricula. This framework is discussed further within the context of clinical supervision (see Chapter 9).

In summary, knowledge of theoretical frameworks facilitates the analysis of communication. It also helps to clarify the purpose of specific interactions. Transactional analysis and six category intervention analysis are examples of theories which have wide application to nursing communication. Both theories serve to simplify analysis and reflection without omitting important issues.

The purpose of the interaction

Whatever the context, a nurse's role is multifaceted. Each facet of the role carries expectations on the part of the nurse and the others involved. The art of nursing is being sensitive to what is required in different situations and responding accordingly. Theories such as six category intervention analysis and transactional analysis are helpful in gaining clarity of the purpose and process of interactions. They are not, however, the full story. The nurse requires the interpersonal skills needed to ascertain data and information and to make a competent response. The other important element is less tangible but involves the ability to build a relationship with others based on sensitivity and understanding (these ideas are discussed in some detail in Chapter 7). When these three elements are integrated into nursing interactions the purpose and consequently the appropriate intervention will emerge.

CONCLUSION

The potential for communication to go astray in nursing interactions is considerable. This has serious implications for all nurses because nursing is essentially an interpersonal process. Research over the last three decades has drawn attention to the importance of effective communication and has called for an increased emphasis on communication in UK nursing curricula. This chapter has highlighted some of the problems associated with nursing communication and suggested some solutions to improve matters. Becoming more effective as a communicator is a process of constant self-development.

This self-development involves several important strands which are detailed in Box 5.6. Combined, these strands can increase the chances that communication will be effective.

Box 5.6 Four strands of self-development

1. Exploiting opportunities to increase awareness of oneself in an attempt to understand others and their experience of us.

2. Learning to use interpersonal skills in a competent, concerted and integrative fashion.

3. Referring to relevant theories in an attempt to analyse, reflect and process interactions.

4. Being clear about the purpose of interactions and matching interventions intentionally.

REFERENCES

Berne E 1966 Transactional analysis in psychotherapy. Grove Press, New York

Boud D, Keogh R, Walker D 1985 Reflection: turning experience into learning. Kogan Page, London

Bradley J, Edinberg M 1990 Communication in the nursing context. Appleton Century-Crofts, Connecticut

Burnard P 1985 Learning human skills: a guide for nurses. Heinemann, London

Burnard P, Morrison P 1991 Nurses' interpersonal skills. Nurse Education Today 11: 24–29

Chant S, Jenkinson T, Randle J, Russell G 2002 Communication skills: Some problems in nursing education and practice. Journal of Clinical Nursing 11: 12–21

Davis H, Fallowfield L (eds) 1991 Counselling and communication in health care. Wiley, Chichester

Dickson DA, Hargie O, Morrow NC 1989 Communication skills training for health professionals: an instructor's handbook. Chapman & Hall, London

Dunn B 1991 Communication interaction skills. Senior Nurse 11(4): 4–8

Egan G 1985 Exercises in helping skills. A training manual to accompany the skilled helper, 3rd edn. Brooks/Cole, Belmont

Egan G 1998 The skilled helper: a systematic approach to effective helping, 7th edn. Brooks/Cole, California

Faulkner A 1985 The organisational context of interpersonal skills in nursing. In: Kagan C (ed) Interpersonal skills in nursing. Croom Helm, London

Hayward J 1975 Information – a prescription against pain. The study of nursing care project reports. Series 2. No. 5. London, Royal College of Nursing

Heron J 1990 Helping the client. A creative practical guide. Sage, London

Hewison A 1995 Nurses' power in interactions with patients. Journal of Advanced Nursing 21: 75–82

Kemmis S 1985 Action research and the politics of reflection. In: Boud D, Keogh R, Walker D (eds) Reflection: turning experience into learning, pp. 139–163. Kogan Page, London

Ley P 1988 Communication with patients – improving patient satisfaction and compliance. Croom Helm, London

Macleod-Clark J 1984 Verbal communication in nursing. In: Faulkner A (ed) Recent advances in nursing 7: communication. Churchill Livingstone, Edinburgh

Menzies EP 1970 The functioning of social systems as a defence against anxiety. Tavistock, London

Meryn S 1998 Improved doctor–patient communication: not an option but a necessity. British Medical Journal 316: 1922–1930

Paggano MP, Ragan SL 1992 Communication skills for professional nurses. Sage Publications, London

Patterson CH 1988 The function of automaticity in counsellor information processing. Counsellor, Education & Supervision 27: 195–202

Peplau H 1988 Interpersonal relations in nursing. Macmillan, Basingstoke

Rogers C 1967 On becoming a person. A therapist's view of psychotherapy. Constable, London

Schon DA 1983 The reflective practitioner: how professionals think in action. Temple Smith, London

Stein-Parbury J 1993 Patient and person. Developing interpersonal skills in nursing. Churchill Livingstone, Melbourne

Stewart I, Joines V 1987 TA today: a new introduction to transactional analysis. Lifespace, Nottingham

Stockwell F 1972 The unpopular patient: the study of nursing care project reports. Series 1, No. 2. Royal College of Nursing, London

Walker D 1985 Writing and reflection. In: Boud D, Keogh R, Walker D (eds) Reflection: turning experience into learning. Kogan Page, London

Wilkinson S 1992 Confusions and challenges. Nursing Times 88(35): 24–28

2

Part 2
Communication in context

6

Communication in groups and organisations

Lynda R. Miller

INTRODUCTION

Man is predominately a social animal with a primary need of other people for his physical and emotional survival. Human groups are the equivalent of the animal herd. From earliest times we know that families lived within larger groups, gaining protection through safety in numbers. Tribal life also allows the division of labour and a sharing of knowledge and skills so further improving the chances of survival for its members. Out of this structure with its obvious practical advantages an interdependence of members develops. Emotional and social bonds are forged and new pairings with new kinship ties result. For each of us the first group experience takes place within our family which hopefully is the provider of almost all that we need to develop in the early years of childhood. However, before very long we must join a variety of new groups in the attempt to meet a whole host of growing physical, cognitive, emotional and social needs (Activity 6.1).

Activity 6.1 Meeting our needs in groups

In the left column list all the groups, formal and informal to which you belong to e.g. family, work, hobby, sport, social. In the right hand column describe what needs of yours are met in each group.

In the developed world we no longer live in tribes; few of us even live within the small community or village setting. Yet throughout our lives we continue to depend upon, and must be able to function in, both a family group and a variety of larger groups or institutions. We learn to cope with the vicissitudes of family life. Then we are required to relate to other children and adults in the nursery or school situation. At some later stage, in order to earn our living, we must work. That work may take place in a hospital, school, factory or a bank but whatever the organisation, it will operate within the same parameters as any other large group of people. During adulthood our needs for affection, social activity and friendship and the drive to find a sexual partner, provide the impetus to join other kinds of groups. We need a social life and our own family, or its equivalent. We may belong to a sports group, social club, voluntary organisation or a choir. Though these groups so familiar to us as part of the modern world, appear superficially to be very different in form and function to the tribal groups of primitive man, in fact this is not so. Systematic studies of these groups confirm that members behave very similarly and that the same dynamics exist there. Therefore our ability to appreciate the value and complexity of group behaviour and to communicate effectively within the groups of which we are a part is as crucial now as it was in prehistory.

Listed in Box 6.1 are some of the advantages which group members and researchers have identified and which you may recognise from personal experience.

THE STUDY OF GROUPS

Interest in group behaviour and the growth of research into the dynamics of small groups began at the beginning of the 20th century. In 1921 Freud published 'Group Psychology and the analysis of the Ego'. This was the first application of psychoanalytic theory to the group situation; knowledge of unconscious mental processes was used to make sense of group behaviour. Psychoanalytic theory as it has developed, remains a legitimate approach to the understanding of group processes. The work of

> **Box 6.1** Potential benefits of groups
>
> The group situation may provide its members with:
>
> ◆ A sense of being accepted and of comradeship.
> ◆ Development of a personal sense of altruism, i.e. a willingness to give of one's self in the service of other people.
> ◆ A feeling of wellbeing and hopefulness.
> ◆ A source of guidance and support in personal decision-making.
> ◆ A source of vicarious learning.
> ◆ Opportunities for greater self-knowledge.
> ◆ Encouragement for the development of social skills.
> ◆ A source of learning derived from their interpersonal actions.
> ◆ Opportunities for self-reflection and self-disclosure.
> ◆ Catharsis, i.e. emotional release which is shared with others present.

Freud, Klein, Bion and other psychoanalysts is used both in therapeutic groups whose aim is to treat emotional problems or enhance self-awareness, and in organisations and institutions with the aim of identifying dysfunction and improving communications (De Board 1995, Jaques 1994, Trist 1990).

During the same period and, in parallel with the growth of psychoanalytic interest, the new social sciences of psychology, anthropology and sociology began to investigate group structure and functioning.

Whereas psychoanalysts are interested in the unconscious mental processes of the group, psychologists focus upon observable and measurable behaviour. Both are interested in the verbal and nonverbal aspects of communication (see Chapters 2, 3, 4) and acknowledge that much of our communications of our thoughts and feelings to others is transmitted without conscious awareness. Psychologists have contributed vastly to our knowledge of group behaviour and their research has shown how groups of people may be influenced both positively and negatively (Cartwright 1959, Kohler 1943, Lewin et al 1939, all cited in Johnson & Johnson 1975). Within psychology several subgroups have developed, focusing upon different aspects of group behaviour – social psychology, the study of interpersonal communication (Asch 1951, Bales 1950 (both cited in Johnson & Johnson 1975), Argyle 1994); occupational psychology, the application of psychological theory in the workplace; organisational psychology, the study of the dynamics of the functioning of a whole organisation or institution (Elwyn 2001, Hirschhorn 1998, West 1994). Each of these specialities has given us both a greater understanding of interpersonal group communications and in some instances, has suggested strategies for altering or influencing group attitudes and responses.

Sociology, the study of human society and its development and function, also contributes to our understanding of how people relate and communicate in the large groups (Parsons 1953, Sprott 1958, Tuckman 1965).

There is now a huge and confusing overlap of published work and training developments stemming from these different disciplines. For example, from mainstream and occupational psychology we have research about effective versus ineffective teamwork (Belbin 1993, West 1994) and leadership skills (Brown 1975, Johnson & Johnson 1975). From psychoanalytic studies, we have descriptions of unconscious defensive behaviours and their effect as they occur within hospitals (De Board 1995, Hinshelwood 2002, Menzies Lyth 1988). Sociologists and psychiatrists have provided us with important insights into the nature of large institutions and their effect on inmate and carer/custodian alike (Barton 1957, Goffman 1961).

Management and specialist human resource training have been developed. Promotion at work to managerial level now carries with it implications for training via universities or other educational institutions. These courses may offer training in group work skills and effective leadership or there may be an increased focus on the dynamics and functioning of large groups or organisations.

This chapter summarises what we have come to know about interpersonal communication within small groups, large groups and the mega group, the organisation. It discusses the dynamics of each in order to equip the nurse with a basic understanding of the kind of groups in health care settings. Only a brief overview of the research studies supporting this knowledge is possible here. What has been included represents that which is most relevant to the practice of nursing.

GROUPS AND GROUP DYNAMICS

At its simplest a group may be described as a collection of people with a common purpose. However, under such a broad definition a football crowd would be defined as a group. Douglas (2000) points out that any collection of people who are aware of each others presence could be described as a group but it is some form of interdependence plus an increase in the mutual awareness of themselves as a group distinct from others, which produces a significant change. Thus a rather transient loose collection of people becomes a more definitive group. Douglas offers a useful table reproduced below in which he identifies a classification of groups based upon various characteristics (Table 6.1; Douglas 2000, p. 16).

Only within much smaller groups of people meeting regularly and engaged in face-to-face interaction, can we see clearly the emerging, and then recurring patterns of communication and behaviour known as group dynamics. These group phenomena, often completely outside the conscious awareness of the group participants, have been studied by analysts, psychologists and social scientists.

Group studies suggest that the optimum size for observation of group dynamics is seven to twelve people. Though there will be evidence of similar behaviours and role adoption in larger groups, it is more difficult to identify the distinct processes and there will be more silent, less-active members.

Table 6.1 Classification of groups by various criteria (reproduced with permission from Douglas 2000)

Criteria	Classification	Characteristics
1. Nature	Natural/artificial	Familiarity and tradition/novelty and suspicion
2. Origin	Created/spontaneous	Conscious intent/generation by pressure of circumstances
3. Leader	Directive/non-directive	Different ideas of the basis of enduring change in human beings
4. Location	Environmental influences	The ethos, structure and management of the organization in which a group is embedded (e.g. hospital, school, etc.)
5. Members	Selection criteria	Principal characteristics of group members (e.g. age, gender, race, problem, availability)
6. Outcome	Group purpose	What the group is set up or adapted to achieve (e.g. learning, support, change, etc.)
7. Number	Size	The effects of large/small groups
8. Throughput	Open/closed	Whether group membership remains the same throughout the life of the group or not
9. Orientation	Approach	The selected theoretical base of the organization/leader/writer
10. Programme	Choice of activity	The principal activity used in the group (e.g. talk, drama, work, discussion, mixed, etc.)
11. Duration	Time factor	The length of group sessions or the length of time the group exists

Membership constancy and the way in which the group is managed influences its development and will either heighten or inhibit the emergence of group phenomena. A closed group has a restricted membership that constantly promotes cohesion, and this results in the emergence of group phenomena, whereas an open group has a membership that alters from one group to the next and this impedes growth. The provision of clear time boundaries so that meetings begin and end promptly at a preordained, regular time and a suitable physical environment exerts a positive effect and group dynamics become more obvious. The physical environment should be conducive to effective communication. Ideally the room chosen should be free from extraneous noise and interruptions, of a sufficient size to comfortably contain the numbers present, private and reasonably comfortable in terms of heating, lighting and ventilation. The seating arrangements exert a surprisingly powerful influence upon group proceedings, therefore consideration should be given both to the way in which the seats are distributed in the room, and the kind of chairs provided. A circular or horseshoe shape maximises the opportunity to make use of nonverbal cues, e.g. facial expression, eye contact and body language. Chairs of the same height allows every one to be 'on the same level', physically and emotionally.

In these conditions where a group of people meet and interact on a regular basis they begin to exhibit certain behaviours, adopt characteristic roles and styles of interaction in that group.

GROUP DEVELOPMENT: NORMS, BOUNDARIES AND PHASES

Fascinatingly, the study of the functioning of any group will confirm similar group processes and membership behaviours. Neither the group's aim, nor its membership alters this. It is irrelevant whether the members are in a study group, a therapeutic group or a work-related group. Whether managing directors of a board, members of the parish council or of a hospital team, the same kind of patterns will occur. Every group establishes codes of conduct, parameters within which the group will function and every group goes through a series of phases in its development. Moreover each one forms a group identity or special character.

Groups, in the course of their development, lay down certain 'rules' governing members' conduct and communications within it. Though very little of this may actually be made verbally explicit, the group as a whole sets and maintains standards which represent the generally accepted codes of behaviour (norms), for instance, what levels of expressed emotion are permissible within the group, what may be spoken about and what topics are to be avoided. These mark out the limits of what is or is not, acceptable within that group (boundaries). Group pressure is exerted enforcing these limits so that members are controlled and brought into line with one another and with the established leader's authority. Because the group norms represent the consensus of group opinion, pressure to conform is extremely powerful. Failure to do so or infringement of these unspoken rules incurs sanctions, which may include reprimand, ostracism or even expulsion from the group. Take the example of a gang of school children who decide that a particular band, or particular shoes are 'naff'. Within that group it is deemed unacceptable to admire the band or to wear those shoes. Failure to conform to the accepted view may bring forth ridicule, contempt and sometimes rejection of the nonconformer. This is a fairly concrete example of an expression of group pressures to conform but in various, subtle forms it will be in operation in every group. Conformity is predominately a condition of group membership.

From its inception the group will pass through a series of developmental phases which, at best, leads to a cohesive structure within which members work as a co-operative team towards the achievement of common goals. Tuckman (1965, 1977) described five identifiable phases or stages in group development as forming, storming, norming, performing and adjourning.

Forming

In the formative stage the group begins to orientate itself, checking out the social code within it. There will be uncertainty, confusion and anxiety, which tend to be manifest in great reliance and dependency on the leader. Members look to an all-powerful leader to take care of them as if they were incapable of taking care of themselves (Bion 1961). Participation is tentative as members try to decide how much commitment to make and what is expected of them. The leader must be sensitive to these needs and permit expression of views, offer clarification of the tasks and explore the expectations of the group.

Storming

In this stage there is a more open and active exploration of views including the expression of conflicts and hostility both between members and the leader whose power is likely to be challenged. There are often issues of control involving feelings of hostility, competition, dominance and rebellion. Because members are attempting to find a place within the group, there is a heightening of anxiety and fear of being excluded or misjudged. Lack of unity is a feature of this phase. This stormy atmosphere is a normal phenomenon in the establishment of any group and if worked through, eventually gives way to the establishment of trust and greater group solidarity.

Norming

This phase heralds a period of cohesion with the development of a group spirit and solidarity. Roles and rules within the group have become established and bonds between members are being forged. There is a sense of belonging and a group identity develops as the group settles down to the task in hand.

Performing

In this phase we see a working group. Cohesion is translated into activity and there is an increase in commitment as individuals accept work *for* the group. The tone of the group is characterised by a more grown-up attitude with conflict being handled more maturely and leadership tasks are more likely to be shared.

Adjourning

In this phase there is a winding down of the group. It is characterised by a reviewing and summarising of experiences both of the task and of the history of the group. Often there is a reluctance to finish and an emotional response to the coming ending which may include a wistfulness and unwillingness to end. Whilst some members may try to prolong the group or may make suggestions for reunions others may cope by attempting to deny its ending. Again there is a clear responsibility for the leader to monitor this process and help the group to come to terms with the impending loss.

Groups differ in their aim; in some the primary aim is social and emotional, in others it is to accomplish some work-related task. Studies suggest that whatever the stated intentions or aims of a group, there will always be a sub- or hidden agenda. These are the unspoken and unacknowledged private aims or desires of the group members. If such aims are running counter to the group's stated task then they will interfere with this, for example where X has an overwhelming need to assume a position of influence in the group. However the hidden agenda is ever present and is by no means incompatible with the accomplishment of group goals. Someone's personal need for power and influence may be extremely useful to the group if handled in the right way.

LEADERSHIP AND OTHER GROUP ROLES

Some groups emerge naturally, e.g. a number of individuals may form an action group in the community, others are formally convened, e.g. to meet some statutory requirement in a health or social services department. Leadership of the group may emerge by common consent, self-selection or formal appointment. More importantly it is the style of leadership which greatly influences the behaviour and attitudes of group members. In turn that has a bearing on the success of the group in achievement of its goals.

Lewin et al (1939) studied the effects of leadership styles on the group of young people. The youngsters were exposed to three differing types of leadership, autocratic, democratic and laissez-faire, the effects of which had a marked impact on the members' behaviour. As the term suggests authoritarian leadership is one in which the leader is indisputably in control, making all major decisions and plans without consultation or negotiation. Authoritarian leadership produced a higher degree of dependence on the leader and a greater degree of self-interest among the members. Aggression and hostility and a tendency to scapegoating was commonest within these groups. The laissez-faire style favours everyone doing their own thing and a relaxed easy-going approach, the direct opposite of the authoritarian style. One would expect this to be very popular with group members but there are drawbacks and frustrations in such a leadership position. In both the authoritarian and the laissez-faire group, a greater tendency towards aggressiveness was a feature. The democratic style which combined clear leadership of the group with power sharing and group discussion in relation to decisions and activities, produced more initiative together with a sense of personal responsibility and more friendliness among members. It would seem the power sharing and delegation of responsibilities within the group made this the most popular style for most members.

Building upon this now famous study of group leadership, subsequent studies into what constitutes effective leadership have investigated permissive, participative and considerate leadership styles versus restrictive, task-orientated styles or directive, socially distant and structured leadership styles. Stodgill (1974) reviewing this work concludes that the democratic style of leadership produces greater member satisfaction in small groups though members in large task-orientated groups prefer authoritarian methods. However the evidence regarding the effects of each on productivity is equivocal. A work-orientated leadership style which favours socially distant, directive and structured leader behaviour with clear role differentiation of members is likely to be the most productive. The person-centred orientated groups with more shared decision-making and concern for members' welfare are appreciated by members and gives rise to a greater degree of group cohesiveness.

What this means in practice is that being effective as a group leader is a highly skilled and complex task. For example a nurse manager might adopt a style of behaviour and an attitude which indicates a wish to be seen as 'the boss', and therefore set apart from the team in certain respects. Such a manager may be firm and very clear about who does what and where responsibilities lie for achieving certain tasks. He or she is clearly focused on 'work' rather than building 'esprit de corp' or making sure everyone in the team is personally content. Another manager may be much more relaxed, invite opinions about how things shall be done and by whom. This manager adopts a warmer emotional tone towards members of the team with acute sensitivity to their personal concerns and needs. Though the second style may be a more attractive one, it does not necessarily lead to greater achievement of goals, that is to say it does not necessarily get the job done more effectively. What is quite crucial to the group in terms of a sense of satisfaction, cohesiveness and productivity is a leader who is able to clearly define his/her role, the task, related expectations and the role of the group members. In other words, it is vital that the leader is able to provide the group with a sound structure or framework in which to operate.

When deliberating how best to lead a group, it is essential to take into account the conditions under which that particular group must perform. For example, in an emergency where quick, decisive action is called for, authoritarian leadership may prove most effective, e.g. in times of war or in a crisis situation. Where there is less urgency and a greater value in seeking consultation prior to making decisions, as in peacetime policy-making, the democratic process favouring member participation is more useful. Thus modern research interest has moved away from the qualities of the leader and more towards the situational approach to leadership styles (Johnson & Johnson 1975).

Within groups who meet regularly for whatever purpose, other roles as well as that of leader may be observed. As a group identity emerges so individuals find a place or identity within it. Some become a 'silent member'; others may habitually adopt a humorous stance, a 'comic member'. A member may constantly question the leadership or decisions taken taking on the role of 'challenger' or even of a 'saboteur'. Subgroups or cliques may form within the group so that certain members 'pair'. A member may act as the able 'lieutenant' to the established leader or be 'bridge-builder' between the leader and the rest of the group. Sometimes one member is seemingly the universal source of considerable dislike, ridicule, irritation or disdain within the group. In this case the role is that of 'scapegoat'. The same person may play out such roles more or less permanently or members may inhabit different roles at different times in the group's history. It is important to be aware of how people come to acquire these positions within the group and the effect it may have on the whole group. The leader needs to be especially perceptive and sensitive to the two-way processes in operation between individuals and the whole group.

GROUPS IN HEALTH CARE SETTINGS

Throughout the National Health Service there are examples of small and large, formal and informal groups, groups where the principal aim is to carry out a work task and those whose main aim is to provide emotional and social support. Box 6.2 has some examples of these.

LOOKING AT HOW PEOPLE IN GROUPS RELATE

Whatever its purpose a group develops patterns of interpersonal communication in order to reach its

---

Box 6.2 Types of groups

Educational, e.g. parent craft groups, student seminars.

Work, e.g. hospital management, planning and policy making groups, ward meetings.

User representation, e.g. groups of lay people whose task is to monitor and give feedback to statutory services.

Therapeutic, e.g. emotional or social problems such as bereavement, addictions.

Support, e.g. for relatives of patients, for ex-patients with disabilities.

Personal effectiveness, e.g. assertiveness and social skills groups designed to enhance confidence and encourage self-development.

Self-help, e.g. groups run by users themselves such as parents of handicapped children for the purposes of fund raising, education and support.

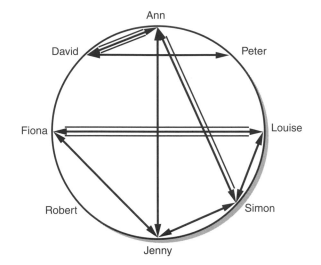

Fig 6.1 Example of a sociogram. Single arrows indicate one-way communication and two-way arrows indicate dialogue

goal. Whether we are present as a participant or a leader, our own responses and the effectiveness of the group in meeting its targets will be influenced by this.

'The co-ordination of information, ideas and experiences and opinions is an essential part of problem solving in a group' (Johnson & Johnson 1975). Getting and giving information is vital to the group's task and the success of the group depends upon the group's culture and each individual's skill in this two-way process of communication.

If we wish to judge how well or ill the group communicates, it is useful to look at communication patterns as they occur. Not just what is said, but by and to whom. Here the focus is upon process rather than content of communications. What is the frequency and length of time each group member speaks? Who speaks to whom and for what apparent reason? Does an individual speak to impress, to win support or to deflect opposition? Who triggers whom in verbal terms? Interruptions give a clue as to the status accorded to members within the group and can be frequently

destructive, damaging and undermining of an individual's contribution.

As an aid to the analysis of group communication, Moreno, a sociologist working in the 1930s, pioneered a technique known as the sociogram (Fig. 6.1). The use of a diagrammatic schema depicting graphically the group's interactions, can be an extremely valuable tool. It has the advantage of avoiding a focus upon what has been said, i.e. the content, at the expense of seeing the pattern in the flow of interactions. After each group the facilitator, group leader and/or co-leader may make a map of the group by drawing a circle representing the group with each member identified around the perimeter. Lines are drawn connecting individuals to indicate the strength and frequency of interactions between them. The emotional tone may also be represented along each line with pluses and minuses to indicate positive and negative exchanges, i.e. degrees of warmth or hostility, supportive versus destructive comments between members. Where seating arrangements are a matter of members' preference, it is useful to notice who sits where and whether this alters from group to group. For example if A sits next to B but is always opposite X, this may have significance and exerts a

Box 6.3 Factors associated with the quality of group communications

Negative factors

Evaluation – a critical, judging attitude
Control – a desire to take over and hold the floor
Strategy – the suggestion that this member is devious rather than transparent in their dealings with others
Neutrality – a non-committal attitude
Certainty – an air of superiority without apparent doubts

Positive factors

Description – ability to express verbally
A problem-solving approach
Spontaneity and openness in dealings with others
Empathy – expressed towards others
Equality – a willingness to share, a sense of fair play

direct effect on the nature and frequency of inter-actions between those particular members. Members often seek out those with similar views or attitudes or those from the same discipline; sitting next to that particular group member may indicate a desire for support or betray anxiety about being in this group. Not infrequently those who are inclined to disagree or who have taken a dislike to each other tend to sit opposite each other in the group, in order perhaps to keep an eye on each other.

The more co-operative a group, the freer the flow of communication between members indicating a willingness to listen to each other, to share and show interest in others' ideas. In contrast, competitiveness within groups gives rise to misinformation, inhibition or deliberate withholding of knowledge and the blocking of the two-way flow of information. A desire for personal power and status tends to make other members more defensive, or to feel threatened or vulnerable. Behaviour associated with a need to look good, to put one over on the others or protecting oneself from attack takes precedence over the accomplishment of the task. It interferes with the ability to accurately perceive the motives, values and emotional content of other group members. This is a significant factor in the loss of efficiency and effectiveness of communications.

Defensiveness also inhibits ability to put across one's thoughts clearly. One member attempting to take control or apparently judging will trigger

defensiveness. This is greatly reduced when communication comes across as an honest desire to find answers to problems, or as predominately helpful to others or is quietly reflective. Most effective are those utterances which imply empathy and concern to the receiver and respect for him or her. On the other hand neutrality in verbal communications tends to be heard negatively. These factors are summarised in Box 6.3.

THREE PATTERNS OF GROUP COMMUNICATION

In a hierarchical group structure communication patterns bear a particular stamp. Such structures are common in hospitals, the armed forces, the public services and in industry. Studies indicate an authoritarian group structure provides a very obvious delineation of tasks, roles and responsibility. In this structure there is a supervisory role so that one member may have responsibility for another or for the whole group's work. This is an arrangement designed to ensure that members fulfil the requirements of them. It is a system dependent upon rewards and sanctions with investment of power in the 'overseer'. It works against power sharing and equality within the group, as unashamedly, it embraces a system in which some members are more equal than others. Communication is formalised, even ritualised, in order to facilitate the achievement of goals, that is to say there are very definite channels for both giving and getting information. In this kind of structure there are expectations of members so that they are required to communicate in a particular way to the designate appropriate senior. It's called 'Going through the official channels'! The structure of the group affects the style and nature of communications within it. The pattern of communication here is predominately one-way.

One-way communication

One-way communication is characterised by the passivity of the ordinary members who are addressed or directed by the chairperson/leader. Questioning or comment is discouraged, e.g. a battalion of troops being given orders. This style has the advantage of speed; it is less frustrating for the leader and more so for the group. Effectiveness of the communications depends on the calibre of the leader in the presentation of the information.

One-way communication with feedback

The one-way with feedback model identified by McGregor (1967, cited in Johnson & Johnson 1975) involves the presentation of the material by the leader followed by an opportunity for questions and clarification with the aim of accurate understanding of the task. The pattern of communication is sometimes known as coercive or directive communication because it is devoid of mutual influence with the assumption that the leader has 'got it right' and there can be no question of any alteration, disagreement or dissent.

In this model and one-way communication there will be considerable frustration among the 'foot soldiers' who often set up informal communication networks of their own in order to sort out the task and clarify their understanding. Many of us will have experienced this in formal learning situations where we became confused but were too nervous or were not permitted to ask for the teacher's help. It is not a very effective method of communication because the informal networks are often faulty with group members disagreeing and growing ever more confused about the task.

Reciprocal (two-way) communication

Reciprocal or two-way communication is the most effective but time-consuming method available to groups. In this system the leader/chairperson sets out to ensure a free flow of dialogue between themselves and the group. Full participation of members is the aim here. In a hierarchical group the leader may implement this form of communication but the particular group structure tends to mean they will still do most of the talking and take ultimate responsibility for the decision-making and actions taken.

TEAMWORK: HOW TO GET THE BEST FROM A TEAM

A work group depends for its success upon the members pulling together. Productivity is not merely a function of shared goals or individuals' technical know-how. Good teamwork depends on effective interpersonal relationships within the group. There has to be a will towards mutual benefit, a sense of being in this together, of mutual obligation and responsibility among team members. 'United we stand, divided we fall' could easily be the motto.

A team's effectiveness can be analysed and evaluated. Ideally these data provide a basis for improvements in individual performance, greater co-operation between team members and improved productivity.

Although work groups are convened for the primary purpose of sharing information, skills and decision-making in order to 'get the job done', it has been proved that group dynamics are still going to be very much in operation. Because group members are often only partially conscious, and sometimes totally unconscious, of group processes, these undercurrents may work for or against the

Box 6.4 Checklist (after Hardingham & Royal 1994)

Productivity – Is the group doing enough? Is there a sense of dissatisfaction with progress?

Empathy – Do members feel comfortable with each other? Is there a tense atmosphere at meetings?

Roles and goals – Do members know what is required of them? Is there confusion about priorities?

Flexibility – Are members open to new/ alternative ideas and contributions? Is there a rigid adherence to procedures?

Openness – Do members say what they really think? Is there a lack of meaningful debate?

Recognition – Do members praise one another and acknowledge achievements? Is there backbiting and sarcasm?

Morale – Do people want to be in this group? Where did everybody go?

achievement of the stated group aims. It is important to understand how groups can be facilitated, how they may malfunction or even cease to function at times as a result of these processes. A better understanding of our own feelings and behaviour within a group is likely to enhance our effectiveness within it. A group leader needs to develop the appropriate insights and skills so that what is unconscious and likely to hamper the group's task is made subtly overt and conscious. Where group members come to realise and appreciate the part played by the unconscious in groups, they are able to be more reflective and more open and honest in their communications. This, in turn, as we have seen, leads to fuller participation of members. The team leader may achieve this in a variety of ways such as via sensitivity groups, team-building exercises and gaming techniques. (See Box 6.4 for some questions we might ask in order to decide how effectively a group is functioning.)

Researchers have considered yet another aspect of the team leader's task, namely the way in which their team interacts with other groups. For instance it may be useful in the health services to consider the way in which one department or discipline relates to another, e.g. the acute services relationship to the rehabilitation area or community care services, the medical staff to nursing staff.

Ancona and Caldwell identified three strategies or predominant patterns which teams use in the management of their boundaries when dealing with other groups within their organisation (cited in West 1994).

1. Ambassadorial activities, i.e. networking with the aim of influencing senior management. This promotes the team's profile and provides senior management with an image of an effective, committed and innovative team. It also secures organisational resources and protects the team from excessive interference.

2. Task-coordinator activities which improve communication with other teams and departments. This activity focuses on coordination, negotiation and feedback across the organisation, i.e. with groups working in parallel to their own.

3. Scouting activities whose aim is to provide the group with up-to-date information on requirements and on developments. These activities are designed to make the team aware of the relevant changes occurring in the external environment, e.g. comparison with other organisations or similar groups, contact with researchers and perusal of journals.

Teams may employ one, all or none of the above strategies, but teams which employed all three had the highest score of all in team performance, cohesiveness and task processing. Co-operation between groups is required by organisations even when they are in competition for resources, e.g. finance or office space. Research confirms that co-operation works better than competition and is more productive. There is a strong case for multidisciplinary or cross-team collaboration as it does generate greater creativity and innovation (West 1994).

Teams need to find creative ways of working which challenge existing orthodoxies substantially. Such creativity only comes from constructive conflict and a preparedness to tolerate and even encourage uncertainty and ambiguity. In this way those who work in teams can experience the excitement of mutual collaboration. If the motivation and commitment of people are to be engaged, there must be a strong sense of the value of the work they do whatever the remit.

This research, though carried out in an industrial setting, is undoubtedly valuable and relevant to the improvement of any team's performance in whatever setting, including the NHS.

SUPPORTIVE GROUPS

So far discussion has been directed at groups with a work or educational task where understanding and analysis via a behavioural or systemic psychological approach is often chosen as the most appropriate and least time consuming. After all, the primary aim is one of conveying information or skills effectively, not greater self-knowledge, personal contentment or alteration of individual attitudes. Educative groups can also be emotionally supportive but this is a spin-off effect as opposed to the primary aim of insight, attitudinal change and emotional support of a therapeutic or support group. For example, in antenatal and postnatal work mothers are helped to cope with the demands of their new role, practically and emotionally.

In supportive groups the remit is different because the focus is upon feelings and attitudes. The leadership style and use of psychological theories varies considerably and usually it is the group's aims and the leader's background that tend to determine the methods used. Support groups are valuable for patients with a particular handicap or illness, which carries with it emotional strain and an adjustment of life style, e.g. a disability/dysfunction following major surgery, chronic conditions such as diabetes mellitus or multiple sclerosis. People exposed to loss of a loved one, of parts of their own body or of some function of it, may find it helpful and encouraging to meet with others who are facing the same difficulties and may find ways of dealing with the emotional, social and practical implications.

Groups such as those offered in hospice settings or within voluntary or statutory organisations may help relatives. Carers coping with conditions like Alzheimer's, AIDS or leukaemia are emotionally supported as well as learning more about how to manage their relative's illness practically. Staff groups can provide support where the work is particularly challenging or distressing, e.g. hospice work, paediatrics and psychiatric areas.

Nurses may be required to initiate or lead support groups or take part in treatment groups offered in specialist areas. It is part of the nurse's responsibility to be aware of the existence of such groups in order to encourage or direct patients or relatives if appropriate.

Using the information contained in Activity 6.2, consider how you would convene and manage this patient group.

Activity 6.2 Setting up a support group

Jenny is caring for her son who has severe learning disabilities and is also physically disabled. She has recently met some other carers who are in a similar position. As there is no local voluntary group, they want to set up a group themselves. They would like to get together with others who are caring for handicapped youngsters to pool knowledge, support each other and have social contact. The hospital managers make a room available and suggest you help the carers to establish a support group. Eight people will be joining this group, and you are required to write a short report to your manager outlining the way in which the group will be set up.

1. Include in the report the practical arrangements and needs of the group, the aims of meetings suggesting times and frequency.

2. How might you encourage members to get to know each other and to form a cohesive group?

3. Describe how you as the formal leader of the group would promote and encourage group activities.

4. Discuss ways in which you might promote the use of other resources locally or nationally.

THERAPEUTIC GROUPS

Following on from Sigmund Freud's influential work (1921), clinical interest in group behaviour grew and psychiatrists began to use groups as a means of treatment. Making use of group processes as a means of influencing thinking, feeling and behaviour gained importance and was used by physicians and psychiatrists to treat survivors of both world wars both here and in America (Main 1989). Group psychotherapy techniques became more widespread in psychiatry from the 1940s and a number of eminent psychoanalysts and psychotherapists published their clinical work using therapeutic groups (Agazarian & Peters 1995, Bion 1961, Ffoulkes 1991, Yalom 1995). The Institute of Group Analysis in London provided the first formal analytic group training.

In the 1960s there was a growth in interest in the newer group therapies based upon gestalt, transactional analysis, and humanistic psychological theories. Nowadays many organisations offer training in a variety of group work techniques to doctors, nurses and social workers as a means of treating neurotic symptoms and social dysfunction. The major difference between the psychoanalytic and other schools of group work lies in the way in which the group is run. In the latter members are often asked directly to communicate their thoughts and feelings and may be encouraged to participate actively in exercises designed to help them focus upon their feelings or thoughts in relation to a particular area of their functioning. Activity 6.3 is an example of a gestalt group exercise.

Activity 6.3 Gestalt group work exercise

In this exercise each group member draws a tree using coloured crayons.

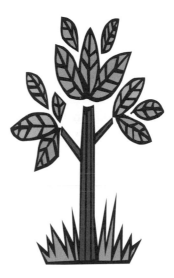

Each in turn then shows their drawing to the group and the leader invites every member to make an observation of that drawing. After everyone has commented, the 'artist' is asked to take a closer look at what they have drawn and is asked the question, 'How might this tree be a bit like you?' This is a prompt to say how the drawing could perhaps be a reflection of how they are, or how they feel about themselves. In this drawing, given there is no evidence of roots, the member may talk about not feeling as if they have 'roots' anywhere. The leaves are full and green so it may be that they talk about feeling good and healthy or particularly productive at this point in their life.

Now find a friend or colleague with whom you feel at ease and each of you draw the kind of house you might like to live in. Making use of the same techniques described in the tree exercise discuss what you have each drawn. Focus not only on the kind of house you or your partner have drawn but also use it to think about yourself, your life and ambitions for the future, etc.

This kind of exercise helps to break the ice between members and encourages openness about one's self within the group. It is also designed to heighten perceptions, promoting discussion and greater self-awareness.

However, therapeutic groups where the aim is to exert a positive effect upon an individual's state of mind and influence behaviour, tend to be conducted by those with a psychodynamic, or psychoanalytic background. The group leader has an interest in the unconscious processes at work within the group. He or she is less active and adopts a more nondirective approach than those common to other therapies. Some group leaders focus on each individual's communication, some reflect and interpret in terms of the whole or collective group's behaviour and communication. All are dedicated to making conscious the unconscious and often unhelpful, forces at work within the group in the interest of promoting a change in individual attitudes and functioning.

In the 1960s when closure of the long-stay psychiatric and mental handicap institutions began, the field of social psychiatry developed. Group work began to be used as a therapeutic agent in both acute inpatient areas and in day hospital and other community-based settings. It is used to treat a variety of psychiatric symptoms and to help in the re-integration of individuals back into society.

In corrective establishments and special units where the aim is to alter aberrant behaviour, group treatment has been used for many years, e.g. Grendon Underwood Prison, The Faithful Foundation for the treatment of sexual offenders, The Henderson Hospital. Applying the principles of group dynamics to the running of the whole community and using groups to examine the nature and effect of individuals' behaviour on others was pioneered by a psychiatrist, Maxwell Jones who coined the term 'therapeutic community'. Such units help people whose behaviour is damaging to themselves or others, e.g. violence, delinquency, drugs or alcoholism, self-harming and suicidal behaviour.

THE ORGANISATION: A VERY LARGE GROUP

Organisations are large groups or, more precisely, they are collections of groups or teams, within a larger group. All that we have come to know about teamwork, leadership and group communication is pertinent to the understanding of the dynamics of the factory, educational institution, large corporation, hospital or a community health facility. The NHS, the largest employer in Britain, has provided social scientists with fertile ground for research into both the dynamics of groups and the large organisation, not merely as an academic exercise but in an attempt to improve efficiency and reduce staff wastage. Within this vast institution, nurses are the biggest professional group. Frequently the nurse is part of a multidisciplinary team which may have a therapeutic, educative or management aim. Once qualified they often find themselves in key position perhaps as a leader of one or more of these groups. As such, there is an expectation that they will get a certain job done as effectively as possible within a time constraint. The leader, whether as a very senior manager or head of a shift, is also responsible for maintaining staff wellbeing and morale. Familiarity with group psychology and with the most recently published work regarding effective teamwork and the specific dynamics of health care institutions is invaluable as it is liable to encourage useful contributions and lessen stress.

ORGANISATIONAL AND GROUP DYNAMICS SPECIFIC TO HEALTH AND SOCIAL CARE SETTINGS

Interest in how health care organisations deal with the vast attendant anxieties generated as a result of the task of providing medical, nursing and social care began with the publication of Isabel Menzies' book, 'Containing anxieties in Institutions' (1988; see Chapter 1). She, like a number of her colleagues from The Tavistock Clinic and the Tavistock Institute of Human Relations, began to apply psychoanalytic understanding of human beings to the form and functioning of health care organisations. This work undertaken over the past 40 years has been dedicated to asking the following questions. Where do anxieties spring from? In what way does the organisation attempt to manage them? In what way does this affect communication and relationships within the ward or hospital concerned? By what means might the stress levels in such situations be improved?

Like Menzies, Obholtzer and Roberts (1994) also use their psychoanalytic background to make sense of 'particularly anxious institutions in the health and social service organisations' but with the addition of Systems Theory drawn from mainstream psychology. Here the group is viewed as a 'system', a social system which makes use of the members' collective energies and resources (inputs), to produce an end product. The end products are the activities and the achievements of the members. Since these end products are rewarding to members, they also provide a source of renewal of energies towards further activity and goal achievement. This cycle is seemingly self-sustaining but of course members receive all kinds of input from outside the group which will contribute to their willingness and ability to sustain efforts on the groups' behalf.

Obholtzer and Roberts have developed a consultancy group service providing a consultant who may be called in as a trouble-shooting expert. They are especially interested in authority and leadership roles as key aspects of organisational life. The consultant's aim is to bring about change by focusing on those members within the organisation who have authority and can be agents for change. Being an 'external resource her/himself the consultants attempt to introduce new perspectives in thinking. S/he concentrates upon the management system within the organisation, focusing upon the task of the institution, its boundaries and the exercise of authority and leadership'.

Hinshelwood and Skogstad (2002), published a number of studies of organisations providing health care. Taking a less active position than Obholtzer and Roberts, they adopted an observational role and deliberately refrained from intervening in any way. (This may strike the reader as odd if one is hoping ultimately for improvements or some positive outcome. It is a position borrowed from psychoanalytic work where it has been long recognised that there is a positive influence exerted by a benign, noncritical presence.) From this standpoint Hinshelwood and Skogstad argue that as insiders they were better placed to understand both the nature and culture of the particular organisation. As participant observers they noted that this kind of work generates huge and often unmanageable anxiety, which the whole organisation has to contain and defuse. Hinshelwood and Skogstad describe three major sources of anxiety and distress to which health professionals are subject:

> First of all, specific kinds of anxiety are connected with particular forms of work. Secondly, the people drawn to particular professions and certain fields within them are usually people with certain kinds of personal anxieties and defence mechanisms, and this in itself has a strong influence on the culture. Thirdly, there are very different ways of dealing with these general and personal anxieties with an organisation leading to different kinds of culture. (Hinshelwood & Skogstad 2002)

In the first instance, for example, working with people who are suffering physically and likely to die puts us in touch with all kinds of personal fears, concerns about our capacity to heal, anxieties about hurting or damaging others and fears about our own death and capacity to bear physical pain.

Then people may be drawn to a particular area of work in line with deeply personal and perhaps totally unconscious needs or anxieties. It may be that the oncologist lost a family member who suffered from cancer; the midwife may have strong feelings about motherhood and babies bound up with her personal longings; someone in doubt about their own cleverness may choose to become a tutor or to work with the learning disabled. Each individual brings to their work their own very personal and particular anxieties, e.g. the need to 'make better, to be seen as a good or worthwhile person or to achieve highly in their professional life'.

People choose, much more than they are consciously aware of, the kind of work they will do. Hinshelwood describes the difference in the types of strain which result from working in obstetric, psychiatric or geriatric specialities. Moreover he reminds us that the work we do may fit in very well with our own habitual ways of dealing with anxieties. For example those of us who cope with unconscious anxieties by organising and cleaning up in our external world, may well choose a speciality which relies heavily on meticulousness, for example in the operating theatre.

In the last statement there is a suggestion that the group as a whole (the organisation) exerts an influence on the individual via the established and generally accepted ways of dealing with distress. The norms of the group or the culture system of the institution or professional group play a part in how individuals respond. Thus individual workers response to the anxieties generated by their work is also heavily influenced by the messages put out by the institution in which they work.

'The third shaping influence of anxieties and defences on the culture is the collectivity of the individuals as they adjust or distort their work practices. These vary from organisation to organisation and with them the way anxiety is "contained" within the culture.' (Hinshelwood & Skogstad 2000). The atmosphere within an organisation is a crucial factor in the unconscious responses of the individuals working there. For example in areas where mortality rates are high 'the relentlessness of death seemed to provoke a similar relentless process of dealing with it'. In the acute cardiology ward the staff exhibited a 'stoical brightness', and this brisk cheerfulness served to hide the unconscious pain of helplessness in the face of mortal illness. Attention is drawn to the negative aspects of this where patients, relatives and less-defended staff members may be more realistically in touch with the emotional pain of their loss.

From such studies we know that without insights into the institution's functioning, care is less effective and staff loss high. Currently there is a crisis in nursing simply because so many have left the profession. In health and social services the main resource is people and the end product is a healthier happier person. An understanding of how people relate to one another within groups, how they may be either supported or further distressed by the groups in which they must inevitably function is crucial and central to our task as nurses or as managers of human resources.

CONCLUSION

This chapter introduced the concept of groups and group dynamics and the functioning of the large group or organisation with particular reference to the work undertaken in hospitals and long-stay care institutions. However only by active participation in groups can we develop group work skills and real insights into group behaviour. By becoming part of a group and reflecting upon it in the company of the other members we discover the subtleties of the working of groups. You may be interested to look at some of the techniques used by group facilitators described in books listed in the Further Reading section.

Effective group communication skills and a knowledge of group relations is essential to the professional nurse in the modern day health and social care services. Whatever their level of training or chosen area of work, the nurse must be able to make use of the power and influence of groups in their roles as clinician, educator and manager.

REFERENCES

Agazarin Y, Peters R 1995 The visible and invisible group. Karnac, London

Argyle M 1994 The psychology of interpersonal behaviour. Routledge, London

Argyle M 1995 Social psychology. Longman, London

Barton R 1957 Institutional neurosis. Wright, Bristol

Belbin MR 1993 Management teams; why they succeed or fail. Butterworth-Heinemann, London

Bion W 1961 Experiences in groups. Tavistock, London

Brown R 1975 Group processes. Blackwell, Oxford

De Board R 1995 The psychoanalysis of organisations. Routledge, London

Douglas T 1988 Basic groupwork. Routledge, London

Douglas T 2000 Survival in groups, 3rd edn. Open University Press, Buckingham

Elwyn G 2001 Groups. A guide to small group work in healthcare, management, education and research. Radcliffe, Abingdon Oxon

Freud S 1921 Group psychology and the analysis of the ego. Volume 18, Standard Edition. Hogarth Press, London. Reprinted 1978

Ffoulkes SH 1991 Group analytic psychotherapy; method and principles. Karnacs, London

Goffman I 1961 Asylums. Penguin Books, Harmondsworth

Hinshelwood R, Skogstad W 2002 Observing organisations – anxiety, defence and culture in health care. Routledge, London

Hirschhorn L 1998 The workplace within, psychodynamics of organisational life. MIT Press, Boston, MA

Homans GC 1958 The human group. Pelican, Harmondsworth

Lewin K, Lippit R, White L 1939 Cited in Johnson D, Johnson F 1975 Joining together. Prentice-Hall, New York

Jaques E 1994 Human capability, study of individual potential and its application. Karnac, London

Johnson DW, Johnson FP 1995 Joining together, group theory and group skills. Prentice-Hall International, NJ

Main T 1989 The ailment and other psychoanalytic essays. Karnac, London

McLeish J, Matheson E, Park N 1993 The psychology of the learning group. Hutchinson University Library, London

Menzies Lyth I 1988 Containing anxiety in institutions. Free Association Books, London

Obholtzer A, Roberts VZ 1994 The unconscious at work. Individual and organisational stress in the human services. Free Association Books, London

Parsons T 1953 In: Sprott WJH 1958 Human Groups. Pelican, London

Sprott WJH 1958 Human groups. Pelican Books, London

Stodgill L 1974 In: Johnson DW, Johnson FP 1995 Joining together, group theory and group skills. Cited in West M 1994 Effective teamwork. BPS Books, Leicester

Trist E et al 1990 The social engagement of social science – Vol. 1. Karnac, London

Tuckman BW 1965 Developmental sequence in small groups. Psychological Bulletin 63(6): 384–399

Tuckman BW, Jensen MAC 1977 Stages of small group development revisited. Group and Organisational Studies 2: 419–427

West M 1994 Effective teamwork. BPS Publications, Leicester

Yalom I 1995 The theory and practice of group psychotherapy. Basic Books, New York

FURTHER READING

Brandes D, Phillips H 1997 Gamesters' handbook, 140 games for teachers and group leaders, Vol. 1. Hutchinson, London

Brandes D, Phillips H 1982 Gamesters' handbook, Vol. 2. Hutchinson, London

Brandes D, Norris J 1998 Gamesters' handbook, Vol. 3. Hutchinson, London

Johnson DW, Johnson FP 1995 Joining together, group theory and group skills. Prentice-Hall International, USA

Remocker L, Storch P 1988 Actions speak louder. Tavistock, London

Tamblyn D, Weiss S 2000 The big book of humorous training. McGraw-Hill, New York

The counselling relationship

Andy Betts

INTRODUCTION

Most nurses and midwives are not counsellors but are professional helpers whose work includes, to a greater or lesser extent, providing psychological support to people who are experiencing a diversity of personally significant life events. This specific type of communication forms the focus for this chapter which examines the nature of the counselling relationship.

There is some evidence to suggest that many nurses have difficulty in establishing and maintaining a facilitative relationship (Burnard & Morrison 1991, Macleod Clark 1985). This chapter looks at the principles of counselling which health carers may apply to help them become more effective at establishing, maintaining and ending facilitative relationships. It also recognises the importance of developing the ability to continually reflect on these interpersonal encounters. It is hoped that the issues raised will promote a re-evaluation of the reader's own experiences and a clearer sense of purpose, intention and direction in this type of helping.

CLARIFYING THE TERMINOLOGY

Harris (1987) notes that counselling has become a vogue term with a broad populist meaning covering a range of different activities. In contrast to this general meaning, counselling today has a more precise definition within a confined and specialist arena. The counselling movement in the United Kingdom has evolved over the past 40 years to be gradually accepted as a profession that is shaking off a lingering image of well-meaning, untrained do-gooders. Counsellors now have an established professional body – the British Association for Counselling and Psychotherapy (BACP) which is energetic in debating and establishing accredited standards of practice and training for counsellors. It is largely due to these efforts that the term counselling has come to mean a more specialist form of helping. Despite this maturation, Howard (1988) questions whether it is possible to write a definition of counselling which is not 'banal, question-begging or vacuous'. The BACP (2002) defines counselling as follows:

The overall aim of counselling is to provide an opportunity for the client to work towards living in a way he or she experiences as more satisfying and resourceful. The term 'counselling' includes work with individuals, pairs or groups of people often, but not always, referred to as 'clients'. The objectives of particular counselling relationships will vary according to the client's needs. Counselling may be concerned with developmental issues, addressing and resolving specific problems, making decisions, coping with crisis, developing personal insight and knowledge, working through feelings of inner conflict or improving relationships with others. The counsellor's role is to facilitate the client's work in ways which respect the client's values, personal resources and capacity for choice within his or her cultural context. (BACP 2002)

This somewhat lengthy definition is the result of much debate and serves to illustrate the difficulties of pinning down what the activity of counselling is in a precise sense. Some of the misunderstandings associated with the term counselling are illustrated by Box 7.1.

There is often confusion regarding the respective meanings of such terms as counselling, use of counselling skills and psychotherapy. This confusion is illustrated in the case of health care workers (see Box 7.2).

Box 7.1 Commonly held myths about counselling

1. Counselling is predominantly concerned with giving advice.
2. Counselling is just common sense – we do it anyway.
3. Counselling is to do with discipline.
4. All health carers are trained in this work.
5. Counselling is by nature vague, unstructured and lacking direction.
6. People can profitably be 'sent' for counselling.
7. Nurses do not have time for counselling.
8. Counselling is about talking, not action.

Box 7.2 Counselling or the use of counselling skills?

Kathy, a staff nurse on a children's ward listens skilfully to the mother of a 5-year-old child who has been admitted for minor surgery. Kathy allows the mother to express her fears about the operation without intruding or belittling them. In everything that she does and says Kathy demonstrates genuine concern for the mother as she tries to understand from her perspective.

At this time is Kathy engaged in listening skills or counselling skills or counselling, and does it matter? The BACP (2002) states clearly that unless both the user and recipient explicitly contract to enter into a counselling relationship then the helper is using counselling skills rather than counselling. If we observed Kathy in both a contracted and non-contracted counselling relationship, she may do the same thing in both situations. Therefore, an important distinction is whether the counselling is explicit or not. In this example if Kathy and the mother had not openly contracted counselling then Kathy was using counselling skills rather than counselling. For most health carers in the majority of situations this is likely to be the case.

To complicate matters further it can be argued that the skills Kathy demonstrates are not exclusively 'counselling skills' but are interpersonal or communication skills which are widely applicable in many other contexts for many different purposes (Bond 1989). Certainly the skills learned in becoming a counsellor are lifeskills in as much as they equip the individual for most other human encounters. Perhaps there is no clear demarcation between these various activities and, as suggested by Pratt (1990), the differences being searched for are more to do with the definition of roles than those of practice.

The ethical importance of this discussion is to protect the client by ensuring that they are not exploited, deceived or harmed by individuals who do not realise, or who choose to deny, their own limitations. In addition, unless helpers are sure about what it is they are engaged in, it is unlikely that they will know how effective they are.

Counselling and advice

Counselling and giving advice are different types of helping. Advice is given from the helper's frame of reference but counselling is firmly grounded within the client's frame of reference. Advice giving is more directive and consequently takes away some of the self-responsibility of the client. Most counselling approaches are less directive and serve to empower clients to help themselves. Both types of helping have a place in nursing but the wise nurse knows clearly when advice is appropriate and when to use counselling skills.

Counselling and psychotherapy

A long-running debate continues on whether a difference exists between counselling and psychotherapy and if so, what it is and is it helpful? There is a growing consensus that the terms may be used interchangeably in most cases (Patterson 1986). This impetus resulted in the formation of the British Association for Counselling and Psychotherapy in 2000, an organization previously known as the

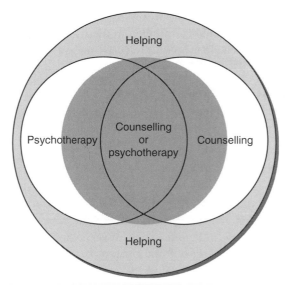

Fig 7.1 Counselling/psychotherapy spectrum

British Association of Counselling (BAC). However, there may be extremes at either end of the spectrum that could not be readily described as one or the other (see Fig. 7.1). Psychotherapy, for instance, is rarely brief in duration whereas counselling is often short-term and may comprise only a few agreed sessions. At the other end of the spectrum, a person attending sessions three times per week for several years and focusing on reconstructive work is unlikely to define this as counselling but as psychotherapy.

So where does this discussion take us and how may it shed light on an understanding of the counselling relationship in the context of health care?

Confusion about the term counselling probably exists because of the word's historical associations. The term 'to counsel' has been interpreted by many as a catch-all verb covering a whole range of human interactions. Over recent years the definition of counselling has evolved to mean a more specific helping activity. While these two distinct uses of the term co-exist confusion is likely to remain. However, the principles examined in this chapter have some application for all nurses in whatever context because they are engaged in what is essentially a helping and interpersonal process. A minority of nurses who have appropriate qualifications may use more formal counselling in their work but only when this is openly contracted with the client.

THE COUNSELLING RELATIONSHIP

Aims

Counselling comprises hundreds of different approaches with widely contrasting views. Nevertheless, all these approaches share a broadly common aim, i.e. to lead to valued outcomes in the client's day-to-day life. The counselling relationship is not an end in itself but a means to an end. Much as we all seem to value the attention and understanding of another individual this should not be the primary reason for counselling. The counselling relationship is only effective to the degree that it translates into more effective living on the part of the client. As a direct result of the counselling relationship something should happen outside of it. Egan (1998, p. 7) notes:

Helping is about results, outcomes, accomplishments, impact ... if a helper and a client engage in the counselling process effectively, something of value will be in place that was not in place before the helping sessions ... helping is about constructive change. (Egan 1998)

This does not mean that the counselling relationship always ends with the client riding off into the sunset, all dreams fulfilled. Indeed, often the client's experience is a painful and demanding one but the ultimate aim is an improved quality of life. The emphasis of the relationship is concerned with helping the client to manage problems and develop unused opportunities towards living more resourcefully. The goal is not for the health carer to 'solve' the problem for the client but to provide the structure in which the individual is able to do the work and resolve the conflict in her own way (see Box 7.3).

Box 7.3 Aims of the counselling relationship

1. To enable others to live more satisfying lives.
2. To provide an environment which helps others to help themselves.
3. To empower others to live more resourcefully and independently.
4. To assist others to manage their problems.
5. To help others to develop their unused resources and opportunities.
6. To enable others to come to terms with changed circumstances.

To some extent this may cause dissonance for professional carers. There is evidence to suggest that health care professions have a history of taking away responsibility from the client/patient (Stimson & Webb 1975). The counselling relationship involves holding back on doing some of the things that carers do as part of their wider role. The wise adage applies that if you give a man fish he eats for the day; if you teach him to fish he eats for life. In other words, if you provide the space in which clients are able to help themselves they may not need future assistance because they have increased their own personal resources. In this context a secondary aim of health carers in the counselling relationship is to do themselves out of a job! Helpers should not be in the business of maintaining dependence but of empowering others to live more resourcefully and independently. In this sense the relationship is a collaborative partnership which has the client's self-responsibility as a core value.

The nature of the relationship

Being with others

The principles of counselling are illustrated in Figure 7.2. The inner triangle contains the client and represents two important points. First, that the relationship is client-centred in the sense that the helper is there for the client in an unambiguous

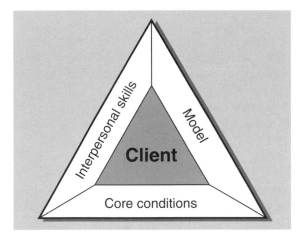

Fig 7.2 Principles of the counselling relationship

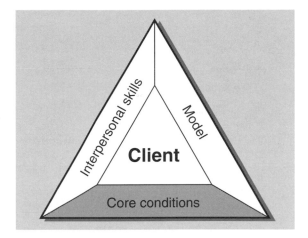

Fig 7.3 Core conditions

way. The relationship is very different to everyday encounters because the helper is there for the client – the dialogue is concentrated primarily on the thoughts, feelings and behaviours of the client. Most other human interactions are characterised by a more symmetrical exchange of mutual interests. Mearns and Thorne (1988, p. 5) underline the principle that counselling is a pursuit of the subjective reality of the client: 'High value is placed on the experience of the individual human being and on the importance of his or her subjective reality.'.

Second, the helper holds and contains the structure and space in which the client does the work. The helper, represented by the external triangle of the diagram, contracts to hold a safe space for the client, represented by the inner triangle. This space consists of more than just the physical environment in which the counselling takes place. It also refers to a therapeutic space which represents a 'safe island' that is distinct from the rest of the client's experience. This space has clear boundaries that are established and maintained by the helper. The client experiences the helper as strong enough to both protect these boundaries and to not be overwhelmed by what the client brings to the session. Put simply, the helper is responsible for the process and the client for the content.

It is not by chance that the core conditions form the base of the triangle (Fig. 7.3). They are the

foundations on which the counselling relationship is established, maintained and ended. Counselling is often described as a way of being with another person rather than a series of behaviours. This emphasis on the values of the relationship has much of its origin in the work of the humanist psychologist Carl Rogers (1951, 1967). He focused more on the qualities of the relationship itself than on the strategies, skills, techniques, models and frameworks being used by the helper. There is general agreement with Rogers' view (1967) that these core conditions are a necessary requisite for meaningful helping to take place but less consensus regarding his belief that they were sufficient in themselves.

The challenge of exhibiting these values with all clients in all counselling relationships appears daunting (see Box 7.4). Rogers (1967) acknowledges that these qualities are ideals for which the

---

Activity 7.1

Examine the ten questions posed by Rogers (Box 7.4). How many are you able to honestly answer in the affirmative in the context of your own helping relationships? How relevant are they to your nursing role?

Box 7.4 How can I create a helping relationship? (Rogers 1967)

1. Can I *be* in some way which will be perceived by the other person as trustworthy, dependable or consistent in some deep sense?

2. Can I be expressive enough as a person that what I am will be communicated unambiguously?

3. Can I let myself experience positive attitudes towards this other person – attitudes of warmth, caring, interest and respect?

4. Can I be strong enough as a person to be separate from the other?

5. Am I strong enough within myself to permit this person her separateness – can I permit her to be what she is?

6. Can I let myself enter fully into the world of her feelings and personal meanings and see them as she does?

7. Can I be acceptant of each facet of this other person which she presents to me?

8. Can I act with sufficient sensitivity in the relationship that my behaviour will not be perceived as threat?

9. Can I free her from the threat of external evaluation?

10. Can I meet this other individual as a person who is in the process of becoming, or will I be bound by her past and by my past?

helper continually strives rather than consistently achievable standards. All of these core conditions exist on a continuum rather than an 'all or nothing basis'. The lifelong task for the helper is to continually strive to establish relationships based on these core conditions while acknowledging the reality that she will fall short of maintaining these conditions in all helping encounters. The core conditions consist of empathy, genuineness, respect and confidentiality.

Empathy

Empathy is often seen as the most critical ingredient of the helping relationship. Carkhuff (1970) argues that without empathy there is no basis for helping. Kalisch (1971) defines empathy as 'the ability to sense the client's world as if it were your own, but without losing the *as if* quality' (Kalisch 1971, p. 203).

This short definition contains some complex ideas. Empathic understanding is often described as 'standing in somebody else's shoes' but this is not the full story. Imagine how you might feel at the end of a day if you stood in the shoes of each person you meet in your helping role – experiencing their thoughts and feelings. Empathy involves retaining your own separateness while trying to understand the world from the other person's perspective. In order to do this it is necessary to understand the client's world as if you were inside it, attempting to see it with the client's eyes but keeping in touch with your own world. In this way the helper remains in a position to help – to get close enough to the client's experience to make a difference whilst retaining a sense of objectivity in order to hold on to the process and not become overwhelmed.

Empathy is different from sympathy – consider the example in Box 7.5.

The second response stays with Claire's experience in that it more accurately expresses what she feels and does not attempt to deny the emotional pain. It is likely that Claire would feel understood and continue to talk about her experience. This is probably more helpful for her than the initial response which is aimed at making Claire feel better in the short-term and illustrates the difference between sympathy and empathy. If empathy is the primary ingredient of effective helping (Carkhuff 1970, La Monica et al 1976, Truax & Mitchell 1971) it is not unreasonable to expect to see it widely demonstrated in the helping professions. You may decide for yourself whether or not this is the case but there are many reasons why it may not be (see Box 7.6).

It is important that helpers not only understand from the client's perspective but actively

Box 7.5 Empathy with the client

Claire lives in a house with three other women. Despite the fact that they all have some learning disabilities they are able to live reasonably independently. Ahmed, a community nurse, visits on a regular basis mainly to help the women with day-to-day management of the house and to offer support and encouragement. Ahmed has recently been working with Claire in helping her to develop more social contacts outside of the house. She had set herself the goal of attending a local church house group for the first time. During Ahmed's subsequent visit the conversation goes as follows:

Claire: (very upset) *'I'm really disappointed – I was too scared to go. I just couldn't face it.'*

Ahmed: (reassuring voice tone) *'Never mind. There's always next week. You will be feeling better by then'.*

Ahmed's response comes from a position of caring and goodwill but is sympathetic rather than empathetic. He fails to acknowledge Claire's disappointment and speaks from a position of optimistic hope rather than reflecting the reality of Claire's disappointment. A more empathetic and skilled response might be:

Ahmed: (concerned expression) *'This was so important for you and now you feel upset that you couldn't go through with it'.*

Box 7.6 Possible reasons for lack of empathy

1. Helpers may 'contaminate' clients' stories with their own experiences, i.e. distort the client's reality because of their own similar experiences.

2. Helpers may make assumptions about clients' experiences that are unsubstantiated – filling in gaps rather than checking out the facts.

3. Helpers may fail to hear the 'music behind the words' – failing to pick up on some of the more subtle cues (often unspoken).

4. Helpers may not have developed the empathic listening and responding skills necessary to understand and convey that understanding to the client.

5. Helpers may lose concentration or be distracted.

6. Helpers may consciously choose not to hear certain things for fear of being overwhelmed.

7. Helpers may track their own lines of interest rather than staying with what the client sees as important.

8. Helpers may rush to move the conversation along rather than acknowledge what has been said.

9. Helpers may pretend to understand rather than check out what the reality is.

10. Helpers may too readily interpret clients' experiences or give advice from their own frame of reference.

11. Helpers may be sympathetic rather than empathetic.

12. Helpers may be judgemental or biased in their responses to clients.

13. Helpers may take over the conversation by talking about their own experiences, thoughts and feelings.

communicate that understanding to the client through the use of skilled communication. In this sense empathy involves both an attitude and a behavioural component. Helpers enter the client's world through attending, observing, listening and then convey that understanding through responding skills. How much of this core condition relates to an attitude and how much to skills is open to debate. It appears that empathic understanding may be increased by teaching the appropriate skills but it is less clear to what extent an empathic attitude or trait is influenced by educational experiences (Reynolds 1987). Clearly the early emotional experience of earlier relationships with other people

will have a significant effect on the individual's ability to understand the world of others. The healthy psychosocial development of a child involves a gradual abandonment of an egocentric view of the world to be replaced by an acknowledgement of the different subjective experiences of others. If the developing child is unable to achieve this transition it is likely to be difficult for her to empathise with others in later life.

Genuineness

This is sometimes referred to as congruence or authenticity. All three of these terms refer to the helper being consistently real in the helping relationship. Corey (2000) suggests that congruent helpers are without a false front and that their inner experience matches their outer expression of that experience and vice versa. In other words what clients see is who the helper really is. Relating deeply to others is a part of the effective helper's lifestyle rather than a role which is taken on and off. Inauthentic helping may appear as 'plastic counselling', or cloned behaviour learned from a counselling trainer or textbook where helpers mechanistically use behaviours and responses that disguise their own integrity, personality and communication style. It is those very qualities that make the helper unique as an individual which serve the relationship. The nurse who switches into 'helping mode' upon the sight of an individual in distress may be perceived by the client as patronising and untrustworthy. Egan (1998) observes that genuine helpers do not overemphasise the helping role, neither are they overdefensive.

Respect

Respect has been described as the deepest human need (Harre 1980). It is difficult to define what is meant by the term. Everyday use of the word tends to be conditional on qualities, attributes or behaviours of others. A person's professionalism, intelligence or skills may be highly respected. The inference being that if the person stopped displaying that aspect of themselves the respect for her may lessen. In the helping context respect is used in a more unconditional sense. Egan (1990, p. 65) defines respect as 'prizing people simply because

> **Box 7.7** Translating respect into behaviour (Egan 1998)
>
> 1. Do no harm.
> 2. Become competent and committed.
> 3. Make it clear that you are 'for' the client.
> 4. Assume the client's goodwill.
> 5. Do not rush to judgement.
> 6. Keep the client's agenda in focus.

they are human' and later summarises how respect can be translated into behaviour (see Box 7.7). The suggestion is that respect remains consistent and is not influenced by the other person's thoughts, feelings and behaviours. The client's lifestyle may differ considerably from that of the helper and may sometimes clash with the helper's values but the effective helper recognises these differences and does not judge the client for them. This nonjudgemental attitude to the client helps provide a relationship which feels safe, warm and accepting. Once again this presents a difficult challenge to the helper. From an early age individuals are socialised into making judgements about others – 'I like him; I don't like her; I don't want anything to do with him unless he'. A helping relationship requires the helper to suspend this type of critical judgement. If the helper is unable to do so then in all probability she is unable to help that individual and is unlikely to be the most suitable person to continue. Acknowledgement of this represents a strength rather than a failure and requires self-awareness, honesty and sensitivity (see Box 7.8).

If Anna had not addressed her own strong feelings and continued to work with Robert it is unlikely that she would have been much help to him. She found it difficult to see past Robert the abuser and was consequently unable to empathise with him. Many people in Anna's position would have experienced similar feelings to a greater or lesser extent. The important point is that she was able to recognise that this was seriously affecting

Box 7.8 Respect

Anna is the named nurse for Robert, a 30-year-old man admitted to the Acute Mental Health Unit with depression. Anna knows that in the past Robert has sexually abused his 7-year-old daughter. When she is with him she feels a sense of disgust and anger that he could have done such a thing. She works hard not to let this show but realises that because of her feelings she is unable to establish a therapeutic relationship with him. She talks to a colleague about the situation and together they decide that it is inappropriate for Anna to continue to be the named nurse. They discuss ways in which the situation could be handled sensitively without Robert experiencing it as rejection.

Box 7.9 Confidentiality

Richard, a community psychiatric nurse (CPN), has been visiting Yolanda, a 33-year-old woman who was referred to the community mental health team by her General Practitioner because she was depressed. In previous meetings with Yolanda, Richard had not explicitly mentioned confidentiality in their relationship. Yolanda has grown to trust him and assumes that what she tells him is confidential. During a home visit she hesitantly discloses that she has been experiencing suicidal thoughts over the past week. She asks that he does not say anything to the doctor because she is afraid he will admit her to hospital. Richard's assessment is that Yolanda is at risk of harming herself and that he has no option but to reveal this information to the doctor even though he realises that this may damage their relationship. He is honest but sensitive in explaining that he is unable to keep this information to himself and although Yolanda is at first upset, no lasting damage is done to the helping relationship.

Robert's care and that she had the courage to address this. Unconditional respect does not mean that the helper condones the client's behaviour but that she is not there to judge him for it.

Confidentiality

Confidentiality is a fundamental feature of the counselling relationship. Understandably people are unlikely to confide in others unless they have some expectation that what they disclose will go no further. The counselling relationship by its very nature is confidential. On the surface this seems a reasonable premise for the nurse using counselling skills. In practice there are limits to the helper's responsibility in this respect. A nurse using counselling skills as a part of her role is still guided by the Professional Code of Conduct of the nurses' professional body, The Nursing and Midwifery Council (NMC 2002), in relation to confidentiality. If a client is in danger of harming herself or others then the nurse has a duty to break confidence. Dryden and Feltham (1992) stress that the counsellor should make the client aware of the nature and limits of confidentiality at the outset of counselling. This may seem an awkward thing to

do for fear of alarming the client but the alternatives could be more difficult to manage.

Consider the example given in Box 7.9.

It is important that helpers are clear about the nature, purpose and limitations of confidentiality in their work and they are not misleading in the messages that they give to the client in this respect.

COUNSELLING AS A SKILLED ACTIVITY

Whilst the core conditions are the foundation of the counselling relationship this type of helping also involves socially skilled behaviours or interpersonal skills (Fig. 7.4). There is a risk that interpersonal skills may be overemphasised in the sense that they are seen as the helping process itself rather than as at the service of the process. Counselling is much more than the application of a range of skills (Johnson & Heppner 1989). If helping is reduced to a series of microskills used in a disjointed or artificial manner then it is likely to be ineffective. Bond

(1989) argues that it is when these interpersonal skills are laden with the values of counselling that they may be seen as counselling skills.

Helpers who are able to establish a relationship based on the core conditions will be more effective if they are competent in the use of interpersonal skills. The aim is to integrate the skills into one's own style of communicating so that they become natural rather than mechanistic. Chapter 5 addresses some of the issues involved in learning these interpersonal skills. Effective helpers continually reflect on their use of skills and understand that they can always improve the way in which they use them. An in-depth summary of the skills used in counselling is beyond the scope of this chapter and is covered in many other texts (Egan 2001, Ivey et al 1993, Nelson-Jones 1995). The main skills required, however, are identified in Figure 7.5. Effective helpers continually reflect on the counselling process, evaluate their use of these counselling skills and

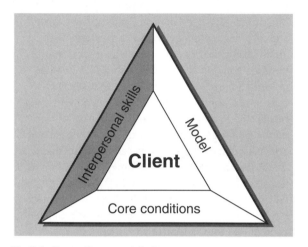

Fig 7.4 Counselling as a skilled activity

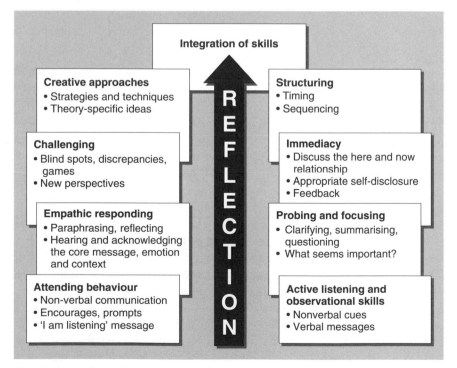

Fig 7.5 Counselling skills

work towards constantly increasing their competence in applying them.

Using a framework

This chapter has suggested that counselling as a specific type of helping is grounded primarily in a way of being with others. Also, that competency in using interpersonal skills appropriately will enhance the effectiveness of the helper. The third side of the triangle (see Fig. 7.6) represents a model of helping. If a helper has access to a model and is able to apply it to these helping encounters then it is likely that the interactions will gain a sense of direction and clarity. A model is a framework which serves the helper by providing a map of the composite territory of counselling. Without this framework or map the complexity of the encounter may confuse or even overwhelm the helper and consequently the client is likely to feel lost too (see Fig. 7.7).

Models in nursing have a chequered history but this may be more to do with the way they have been applied than any shortcomings in the models themselves. A model is only of use to the extent that it serves clients' outcomes. It is not more important than the client and need not be rigidly adhered to in an inflexible manner. Models consist of sets of principles rather than magical formulae and if used wisely enable the helper to make sense of the process and provide direction (see Fig. 7.8).

Karasu (1986) reported finding over 400 distinct counselling and psychotherapeutic approaches, theories, schools, techniques and systems all claiming to lead to success. Since then many other new approaches have become established. To the novice helper this diversity of ideas may appear bewildering and even paralysing in terms of where to start. An alternative way of thinking about these approaches is as a rich source of resources all containing points of merit and potential. Experienced counsellors, after gaining a thorough understanding of the various theories, are able to use ideas from these different approaches and integrate them into their own helping style.

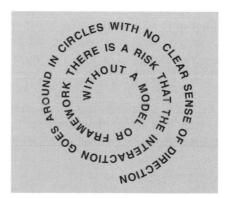

Fig 7.7 Potential difficulty of not using a model

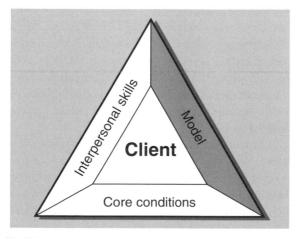

Fig 7.6 Using a framework for helping

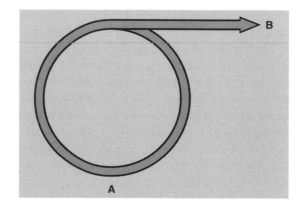

Fig 7.8 A model helps the client to reach a destination

Initially it is wise to learn and become competent with one practical working model or approach. Egan (2001) presents a model called the 'Skilled Helper' which he describes as a systematic approach to effective helping. It provides a pragmatic problem management approach that fits neatly within the process of nursing. It is described in some detail as one possible model which nurses may wish to explore further. The rich diversities of alternative models provide other options if the Skilled Helper does not suit. For example, an alternative approach that is prominently used in health care settings in the UK is cognitive behavioural counselling.

The 'Skilled Helper'

This model of helping provides a practical way of working which is grounded in problem management and opportunity development. Egan (1998) claims the framework enables the helper to structure each step of the change process without ignoring the complexities. There is an emphasis on action that is grounded in the belief that the goal of helpers is to assist others to manage their lives more effectively. Another feature of the skilled helper is that it is integrative in the sense that it enables helpers to use ideas and strategies from the wealth of different approaches within counselling and psychotherapy and to mould them into their own individual helping style.

The simplest and most logical way of describing this model is to progress in a linear fashion through the stages. This enables people to gain a conceptual understanding of the various steps. As helpers attain a behavioural understanding of the model and eventually a mastery of it they are able to use it much more flexibly by smoothly moving around within it. In other words, helping is not a linear process characterised by neat progressive steps; rather it is typically unpredictable and messy. This is why a map is essential to make sense of what is happening without losing the flexibility to respond to the uniqueness of each individual. The reader should bear these ideas in mind when considering the following stages in Figure 7.9.

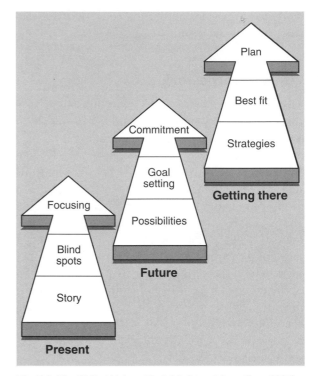

Fig 7.9 The Skilled Helper Model (adapted from Egan 1990)

Stage 1: the present

1.A Telling the story This stage involves the initial exploration and clarification of the situation, issues, problems and opportunities (Fig. 7.10). As discussion progresses the helper is establishing a relationship with the client based on the essential core conditions and the helper's interpersonal skills. By listening to the story, the counsellor gains an understanding of what is going on for the client; through telling the story the client gains some clarity of her situation. A relationship is being established in which the client feels safe and is encouraged to disclose information.

1.B Identifying and challenging blind spots Egan (1998) suggests that most clients need to move beyond their initial subjective understanding of their problem situations. Limited perspectives of their situations may keep clients locked in self-defeating patterns of thinking and behaving. When faced with difficulties we tend to take a tunnel

Stage 1: Present

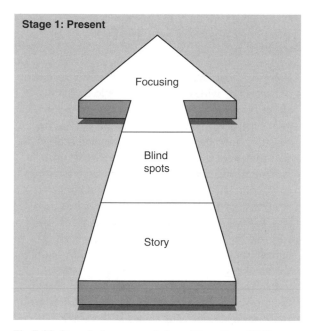

Fig 7.10 Stage 1: the present (adapted from Egan 1990)

Box 7.10 Challenging clients' perspectives

Alison is a student nurse who has recently failed her end of Common Foundation Programme examination. In addition to this a long-term relationship with a boyfriend has come to an emotional end. For some time things seem to have been going wrong in her life and during a tutorial she breaks down in tears. The tutor listens to Alison's story as she recounts her recent life. Alison blames herself for the fact that nothing has gone right for her. She sees nothing positive in her life and talks about herself in terms of a complete failure in relationships, studies and many other aspects of her life. While recognising and acknowledging the pain that Alison is feeling the tutor is able to sensitively point out areas of Alison's life that are successful and strengths and resources which she has demonstrated in her time at the college.

vision of our situations. Challenging blind spots does not consist of invalidating the client's experience or telling them what they are doing wrong. Effective challenging is grounded in empathy but allows the individual to examine alternative perspectives or uncover information that they are selectively disregarding. Examples may include identifying hidden strengths and resources of the client or encouraging them to own their situation or problems. Challenging clients' perspectives is woven into the entire helping process, not just at this stage of the model.

When this challenging is done skilfully and with empathic sensitivity the client is prompted to examine her previously limited perspectives and see the difficulty in a different way (Box 7.10). When done unskilfully with a lack of empathy the client is likely to feel criticised or misunderstood resulting in damage to the helping relationship.

1.C Focusing, screening and finding the leverage Stage 1A explores the present situation. It provides an opportunity for the client to relate a broad and often complex jumble of events, feelings, thoughts

and behaviours. In this format the story is rather unmanageable and so the helper now assists the client to filter out the major themes. This involves screening out the less-significant parts of the story, focusing on the major issues and helping the client to decide which makes sense to work on first, etc. Egan (1998) uses the word 'leverage' to mean the payoff for the client. For instance, the client may come to realise that working on one particular issue will, if managed successfully, contribute to the management of several other related problems. Stage 1C concentrates on breaking down the whole story into smaller, more manageable parts and helping the client to prioritise them.

Stage 2: the future

2.A Possibilities There comes a point when it is helpful to move the client on from talking about what is going wrong to what it is that they want. This stage is concerned with helping the client to look into the future (Fig. 7.11). The question that moves people on is 'what would it look like if it

Stage 2: Future

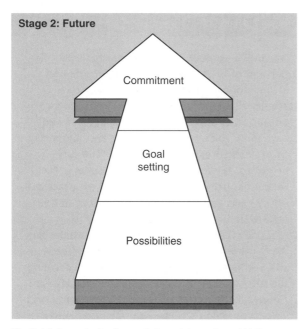

Fig 7.11 Stage 2: the future (adapted from Egan 1990)

Box 7.11 What would it look like if it were better?

Lying in a hospital bed recovering from a recent operation provides time for Antonio to think about his life. In particular he thinks about his relationship with his wife, Maria. He knows they have not been happy for some time and realises that they have both let this situation drift on.

One of the nurses spends some time listening to Antonio and then asks 'what would your relationship with Maria be like if it was just how you wanted it?' This question takes Antonio by surprise but after the nurse has left he finds himself thinking about the kind of relationship he would like to have with Maria. In many ways it is the relationship they used to have and he is able to see what is missing. He resolves to himself to work toward improving things in this way.

were better?' This may seem an obvious question but it is one we rarely ask ourselves when we encounter a problem. More commonly, people find themselves in a problem situation and act before considering how they want things to be different. The fact that we tend not to ask this question of ourselves means that helpers often experience initial resistance at this stage. On the extreme level, a client who is depressed may see no future. If helpers can enable clients to construct images of possible futures for themselves, they are doing something helpful. This stage also helps the process to move forward from what can become a self-indulgent, excessive exploration of how awful the present is. Without such a step the process can go round in circles rather than moving towards outcomes.

Different techniques or strategies may be useful here. For clients who are resistive to this way of thinking, it may prove useful to encourage them to think how it would be if it were a little bit better (Box 7.11). For others fantasy thinking may work, e.g. if you could have whatever you want.... If done sensitively this is not a tantalisation but a strategy to enable the client to realise what is

within the dream that they value for themselves. The art of this stage lies in encouraging the client to free themselves from reality constraints or 'Ah, buts'. The use of creative strategies suited to the individual client is productive.

By asking the question in Box 7.12, the counsellor enabled Steven to rediscover his future. As often happens when people have a terminal illness, others avoid talking about the future. It is as if they have no future at all. By helping Steven to focus on possibilities in his life, the counsellor prompted him to realise what was really important to him and helped him to retrieve a sense of direction and future.

2.B Goal setting Egan (1998) refers to this stage as the 'change agenda' as it prompts the client to move from possibilities to choices. Once the possibilities have been generated by the client, it is timely to help them choose the ones that fit their circumstances. The broad pictures are forged into workable goals. The use of a behavioural checklist at this point may be helpful. Goals are more likely to be achieved if they are stated in terms of the checklist in Box 7.13.

> **Box 7.12** What would it look like if it were a *little* better?
>
> Steven has full-blown AIDS. He sees a counsellor each week and has gradually come to experience these meetings as a safe haven in a world in which he feels unable to talk about what is happening to him. He has found it helpful to express his feelings and talk about his reaction to his changed circumstances. The focus of the interaction has been on the past and the circumstances that led to his situation today. At one of their meetings the counsellor asks Steven *'what is it that you want for yourself?'* This question stops Steven in his tracks and his initial response is rather abrupt *'I wouldn't have this wretched illness'*. The counsellor is able to help Steven to see past this angry response and gradually coaxes him to identify what things he does want for himself that would make a difference to his life. It emerges that he wants to patch up his relationship with some of his family; to increase his support network; to say the things he needs to say to others; to expand his social life. He is even able to talk about his own death and dying and how he would want that to be.

> **Box 7.13** A behavioural checklist for goal setting
>
> | | |
> |---|---|
> | Accomplishment | What will be in place at the end of the day not *how* the client will get there, i.e. stated in outcome terms. |
> | Specific | Describe clearly and precisely what will be in place. Vague statements are unlikely to materialise into action. |
> | Measurable | How will the client know when he/she has achieved the goal? |
> | Realistic | Has the individual the resources to achieve the goal? |
> | Owned | The goal must be the client's goal. He/she is not choosing it to please the counsellor or under pressure from third parties. It should be stated in 'I' terms. |
> | Substantive | Achieving the goal should make a clear difference to the identified problem area. |
> | Values | Is it within the client's values or will he/she find it too uncomfortable to achieve? How may it compromise the client's value system? |
> | Time frame | Many of us live as if we are immortal. We will get round to it someday. Challenging the client to state a realistic and specific time frame for achieving the goal makes it more likely that it will be achieved. |

2.C Commitment Effective helpers leave the responsibility for choice with the clients. They can help the clients commit themselves by helping them search for incentives for commitment. From the identified goals, which are the most urgent and immediate? Also the helper can enable the client to check out the costs and consequences of achieving the goals. For instance 'how much will achieving this goal cost me emotionally?' and 'what will be the effects on others in my life?'

If Stage 2 is done well the client will have a clear idea of what they would like to accomplish, without necessarily knowing how they will accomplish it.

Stage 3: Strategy – getting there

3.A Strategies (possible actions) A strategy is a set of actions designed to achieve a goal and tends to be more effective when chosen from a range of possibilities (Fig. 7.12). If people attempt one strategy and fail they may assume that they will never achieve their goal, or they may try the same strategy again only to fail once more. Suggesting a range of ideas makes it more probable that one or a combination of them will suit the resources of the client. In this step the principle is to suspend

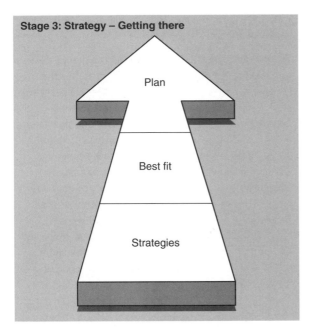

Stage 3: Strategy – Getting there

Plan

Best fit

Strategies

Fig. 7.12 Stage 3: getting there (adapted from Egan 1990)

Box 7.14 Choosing a range of strategies

Rose desperately wants to give up smoking. Her health is deteriorating but all previous attempts to stop have failed. The practice nurse at the health centre offers to try and help. She asks Rose to write down all the possible ways she can think of to stop smoking. With encouragement Rose comes up with the following list:

◆ Join a support group for people trying to stop smoking.

◆ Tell everybody I know that I am going to stop.

◆ Try nicotine patches.

◆ Read books on the effects of smoking.

◆ Reward myself in some way for each day I don't smoke.

◆ Change my social patterns.

◆ Avoid places where others smoke.

◆ Spend the money I would spend on cigarettes on something else.

◆ Avoid shops that sell cigarettes.

◆ Start a keep fit routine to feel the benefits of a healthy lifestyle.

◆ Try hypnosis to stop.

◆ Meet with the practice nurse regularly for support.

◆ Discover things to eat that may replace the craving for cigarettes.

judgement on the ideas (the 'ah, buts') and encourage the generation of as many different strategies as possible. One way of achieving this is to use brainstorming, i.e. not to comment on each idea until after you have exhausted the possible list. Prompting the client to write them down ensures that none get lost in the process.

The helper uses prompts to encourage the client, e.g. the people who may help, the places, the organisations, etc. Often ideas piggyback on previous ideas and sometimes the use of humour or wild ideas is what is needed to get past the impasse to creativity.

Box 7.14 illustrates how by generating a quantity of possible strategies Rose has increased her options. If she had not brainstormed the list with the Practice Nurse then she may have only tried the strategies that had not worked before. Rose probably would not use all of the strategies but would select the ones which best suited her.

3.B Choosing the best strategies The client, in collaboration with the helper, now reviews the different options and chooses the best single strategy or combination. The best strategy or combination of strategies are those which match the client's needs, preferences, resources and are least likely to be blocked by environmental factors. In other words each strategy is reviewed to check whether it is realistic and within the client's values.

3.C Turning strategies into plans The chosen strategies need to be converted into a step-by-step plan which identifies the first task to be done, then the second, etc., i.e. 'putting the flesh on the bones'. This planning should incorporate realistic time frames. The helper's intervention makes it more likely that the client will act and that she will receive support during that action. Remember that the plan is the client's plan, not the helper's. Throughout this model the helper's responsibility is for the process and the client's for the content and decisions. In this way the helper provides the conditions in which the client is able to face issues, make decisions and act on them.

Time spent identifying the possible factors which will either hinder or help the plan is worthwhile. Forewarned is forearmed and the inclusion of contingency plans will minimise the effect of hindering factors and maximise the effect of helpful factors.

The counselling relationship does not usually end here – the helper continues to meet the client to support her and to listen to her progress or lack of it.

An inexperienced helper, and sometimes even an experienced one, may apply the model too rigidly. It is worth stressing here once again that the model is at the service of client outcomes and needs to be managed with flexibility. A framework such as the Skilled Helper can make the process manageable rather than bewildering for the helper and the client.

PRACTICAL ISSUES

When to use counselling

The art of effective helping is recognising the type of intervention that is required for a particular client in a given situation, taking into account their resources. Helping that is based on the values, skills and theories of counselling is only one part of the nurse's role. At other times the helping involves much more directive interactions such as advising, teaching, advocacy, prescribing, etc.

Deciding when a counselling type of intervention is appropriate is a difficult judgement to describe concisely and is as much involved with experience and sensitivity as with clear criteria. In assessing each situation the nurse recognises cues that provide the clues for deciding on the most appropriate type of helping.

Box 7.15 Appropriate helping

Mohamed, a pre-registration Diploma student is on a short placement with a District Nurse. As he observes her working he is particularly impressed with her ability to adapt her interventions to match the needs and circumstances of the clients she visits. On one visit she recognises that a client requires advice and information regarding medication. This is given in a clear and unambiguous manner. The next visit requires a very different interaction as she uses counselling skills to enable a client to express his anguish at the recent death of his partner. Mohamed notices that both of these interventions are skilful and match exactly what the client requires.

The example in Box 7.15 demonstrates that the use of counselling skills is usually one part of the health carer's role. The art of helping is recognising clearly what is required based on sensitivity to the cues which the client provides.

Support and supervision

This type of helping is complex and taxing for the helper. Helpers who take this route pay a price for doing so. The more effective helpers are at this work the more people will open up to them. This can contribute to an increased sense of burden and pressure. The effective helper identifies a clear network of people who provide support and knows how to access this support. Rather than a sign of weakness this represents a strength in the helper. Listening to what may often be painful experiences inevitably stimulates strong emotions in oneself. If these emotions are repressed then the helper is likely to pay the price in the long term. Off-loading to trusted colleagues, co-counselling and support groups are all possible options for support.

Supervision is different to support. Practising counsellors require regular contact with an experienced counsellor who acts as a supervisor for their practice. Although most nurses are not counsellors, the more they use counselling skills in their work the greater the need for this type of supervision. Houston (1990) emphasises that a central task of the helper is to spend time to look again, in the presence of a supervisor, at what the helper and client said and did. The supervisor is primarily there to ensure that the client gets the best possible help from the counsellor. The benefits to the helper are supportive, developmental and educational through reflection on practice. Supervision is explored more fully in Chapter 9.

Safety and ethical issues

This type of helping is not neutral in terms of its effects and can be for better or worse (Egan 1998). Incompetent helpers can damage clients. Kagan (1973) questions whether all counsellors are competent and what happens if they are not. The first rule for the helper is to do no harm and this is achieved by maintaining the core conditions of the helping relationship and by contracting adequate supervision. An important aspect of the counselling relationship is for helpers to realise their limitations and know when it is appropriate to refer on to more specialist help.

Time and resources

A frequent comment from health carers is that they do not have the time to engage in this type of helping. In these days of economic restraint and limited resources the counselling relationship may be viewed as costly in terms of human resources. An alternative perspective is that time spent using counselling skills may actually be less demanding of resources in the long term. If the interaction results in a more accurate understanding of the client's world, self-empowerment and independence, then this may be time profitably spent.

It is of mutual benefit to helper and client if the actual time available is openly negotiated at the outset. Whether this is 10 minutes or 1 hour both parties then know when the interaction will end. This sets the boundary for the client to say what she wants to say and enables the helper to finish the interaction more easily. For those who engage in more formal counselling this time contracting is particularly important and usually includes negotiation of the number of sessions they will meet with the client.

CONCLUSION

This chapter has examined the nature of the counselling relationship in the context of health care, and the communication that takes place with it. Whilst recognising that most nurses and midwives are not counsellors they do provide psychological support to others as a part of their role. The principles of the counselling relationship have application for helpers in this capacity. The foundation of a helping relationship is based on core conditions or qualities, the most significant of these being the values of empathy, genuineness and respect.

Effective helping is also a skilled activity consisting of interpersonal or counselling skills which are underpinned by the core conditions. There are many different models or approaches within counselling and one function of these theories is to provide a sense of direction for the helper. The Skilled Helper is one example of a systematic problem management approach to effective helping that has wide application within health care settings.

REFERENCES

Bond T 1989 Towards defining the role of counselling skills. Counselling 69: 3–9
British Association for Counselling and Psychotherapy 2002 Code of ethics and practice for counsellors. BAC Publishers, Rugby

Burnard P, Morrison P 1991 Nurses' interpersonal skills. Nurse Education Today 11: 24–29
Carkhuff RR 1970 Helping and human relations. Holt, Rinehart & Winston, New York

Casement P 1985 On learning from the patient. Routledge, London

Corey G 2000 Theory and practice of counselling and psychotherapy. Wadsworth Publishers, Belmont, California

Dryden W, Feltham C 1992 Brief counselling: a practical guide for beginning practitioners. Open University Press, Buckingham

Egan G 1990 The skilled helper: a systematic approach to effective helping, 5th edn. Brooks/Cole, California

Egan G 1998 The skilled helper: a systematic approach to effective helping, 6th edn. Brooks/Cole, California

Egan G 2001 The skilled helper: a systematic approach to effective helping, 7th edn. Wadsworth, California

Harre R 1980 Social being. Adams, New Jersey

Harris CM 1987 Let's do away with counselling. In: Gray D (ed) The medical annual, pp. 105–111. Wright, Bristol

Houston G 1990 Supervision and counselling. Rochester Foundation, London

Howard A 1988 The necessities and absurdities of accredited helping. BAC Journal 64: 19–22

Ivey AE, Ivey MB, Simek-Downing L 1993 Counselling and psychotherapy: a multicultural perspective, 3rd edn. Allyn and Bacon, Boston

Johnson WC, Heppner PP 1989 On reasoning and cognitive demands in counselling: implications for counsellor training. Journal of Counselling Development 67: 428–429

Kagan N 1973 Can technology help us toward reliability in influencing human interaction? Educational Technology 13: 44–51

Kalisch BJ 1971 An experiment in the development of empathy in nursing students. Nursing Research 20(3): 202–211

Karasu TB 1986 The spcificity against non-specificity dilemma: toward identifying therapeutic change agents. American Journal of Psychiatry 143: 687–695

La Monica E, Carew D, Winder A, Hasse A, Blanchard K 1976 Empathy training as the major thrust of a staff development programme. Nursing Research 25: 447–451

Macleod Clark E 1985 The development of research in interpersonal skills in nursing. In: Kagan C (ed) Interpersonal skills in nursing: research and applications. Croom Helm, London

Mearns D, Thorne B 1988 Person centred counselling in action. Sage, London

Nelson-Jones R 1995 Theory and practice of counselling. Cassell, London

Nursing & Midwifery Council 2002 Code of Professional Conduct. NMC Publications, London

Patterson CH (ed) 1986 Theories of counselling and psychotherapy, 4th edn. Harper & Row, New York

Pratt J 1990 The meaning of counselling skills. Counselling Journal Feb, 21–22

Reynolds J 1987 Empathy: we know what we mean, but what do we teach? Nurse Education Today 7: 265–269

Rogers C 1951 Client centred therapy: its implications and theory. Houghton Mifflin, Boston

Rogers C 1967 On becoming a person: a therapist's view of psychotherapy. Constable, London

Stimson G, Webb B 1975 Going to see the doctor – the consultation process in general practice. Routledge & Kegan Paul, London

Truax C, Mitchell K 1971 Research on certain therapist interpersonal skills in relation to process and outcome. In: Bergin A, Garfield S (eds) Handbook of psychotherapy and behaviour change. Wiley, New York

FURTHER READING

Egan G 2001 The skilled helper, 7th edn. Wadsworth, California

McLeod J 1998 An introduction to counselling, 2nd edn. Open University Press, Buckingham

8

The mentoring relationship

Patricia East   Roger Ellis

INTRODUCTION

The advent of Project 2000 and Making a Difference curriculum with its common foundation programme and establishment of a qualification with greater academic currency for the newly accredited nurse, makes explicit what was implicit in the past: that entrants to nursing are adult learners. If the nurse needs to be successful as a reflective practitioner in both general and specific areas then the learning environment must match this need.

The curriculum framework for communicating and developing in-depth knowledge of the subject matter and skills required must also be linked to the practice of nursing. The use of mentoring programmes has been widely advocated as a means of providing a developmental bridge between theory and practice for the inexperienced nurse entrant. This chapter examines the conceptual bases for mentoring and its application in organisational, educational and nursing settings.

THE ORIGINAL MENTOR

The Greek poet, Homer, tells the story of Odysseus, King of Ithaca, who, whilst away fighting in the Trojan War, entrusted his young son, Telemachus, to the care of a guardian named Mentor. Odysseus was prevented from returning home for 10 years and the goddess Athena, moved by his plight, assumed the appearance of Mentor to make an earthly visit to stir Telemachus into mounting a rescue operation for his father. Thereafter, Athena would appear in the guise of Mentor whenever she wanted to offer support and guidance.

Athena was the daughter of Zeus and had inherited many of her father's powers and qualities, although she was neither all powerful nor all wise. Often connected with war, Athena was also patroness of arts and crafts, occasionally the goddess of medicine and ultimately the goddess of wisdom. Thus, Athena combined her practical skills with insight and wisdom and a capacity to work on behalf of others.

Modern ideas about mentoring can therefore be seen to have their roots in mythology. Athena could embody both male and female qualities; her purpose was to support and guide others – be they individuals or the state of Athens – to strive for and to achieve the highest goals. In order to do this Athena took the roles of teacher, adviser, counsellor, sponsor and guide, whenever her support was required. She was also able to integrate the needs of the individual into the wider context. This chapter demonstrates how these are all essential qualities for the role of mentor (see Fig. 8.1).

Defining the role of mentor

While it may not be possible to call on a goddess to act as mentor, some definitions of the role are rooted in this classical ideal. Rowntree's (1981) definition of a mentor as a 'trusted and friendly adviser or guide, especially of someone new to a particular role' is drawn from this origin. In this classical definition the mentor becomes involved in a powerful interpersonal relationship with a less-experienced, normally younger person. The relationship involves the engagement of mentor and mentee in the objective and subjective world of each other.

Daloz' (1986) description of a mentor also has classical origins reflected in a Jungian archetypal figure. The mentor represents knowledge, reflection, insight, understanding, good advice, determination and planning; qualities which cannot be mastered alone. Using the metaphor of a journey, Daloz' concern is that the mentor acts as a travelling companion who is more a trusted guide than a tour director.

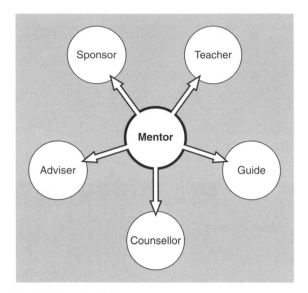

Fig 8.1 The role of the mentor

Daloz refers to the poet Virgil as a classical mentor when he accompanies Dante on his journey through the underworld. This 'mentor supreme' protects, urges forward, explains mysteries, points the way, leaves Dante alone when necessary, translates codes, calms marauding beasts, clears obstacles and encourages – always encourages – helping Dante to find in himself the courage to go on. Embedded in this metaphor is a model for the mentoring role in nurse education. The mentor engenders trust, issues challenges, offers vision, and alternatively supports and challenges the mentee (see Table 8.1).

Virgil knew when to leave Dante, just as mentors eventually need to let go of their mentees. This final point may be linked with Winnicott's (1982) ideas of 'good-enough mothering' and the 'holding environment'. Central to these ideas is the notion that once a child gains a sense of his continuing existence then he is able to successfully separate, initially from his primary caretaker and consequently from others throughout life, without too much anxiety. Kegan (1982) has developed and extended Winnicott's insights across the whole of life-span developmental psychology, describing a procession of 'holding environments' or 'cultures'.

Table 8.1 Dante, Virgil and the nurse mentor

Virgil	Nurse mentor
A well respected authority	A well respected authority
A model poet	A model nurse practitioner
Appears at the outset to offer support, allay fears of isolation, ignorance and ridicule	
Virgil has made this journey before	Nurse mentor has completed her own training and kept up to date with recent developments
Can act as a guide	
Virgil knows the danger spots and can alert Dante in advance – Dante must negotiate the dangers, the pits, the chasms of despair, the cauldrons of boiling blood himself	Nurse mentor knows what lies ahead and can alert her mentee in advance to prepare for the unknown, offer her support and encouragement, challenge and confront when necessary
Can give advance notice and an overview of the whole process, offer support, facilitate learning, give feedback, constructive criticism and praise	
Virgil can understand and speak the languages of the underworld and explain the rules, rituals and symbols to Dante	Nurse mentor understands and can speak in UKCC code and interpret medical terms, academic jargon and the esoteric demands of tutors
Can translate and demystify course requirements	
Virgil explains Dante's quest to the damned	Nurse mentor acts on mentee's behalf
Acts as an advocate	
Virgil leaves Dante at the end of his journey	Nurse mentor recognises mentee's competence
Allows independence and can separate	

Good mentors ensure that their mentees can recognise that authority has its uses but is limited and that the task of becoming independent involves separation from authority figures and taking on one's own authority.

An important introduction to the concept of mentoring can be found in the work of Levinson et al (1978), which examines the contribution of the mentoring relationship over four phases of adult life. According to Levinson, a mentor is neither a parent nor a peer but a transitional figure, usually 8–15 years older than the mentee. If the age difference is greater than 20 years the mentor is likely to act in a paternalistic manner; if less than 8 years then it is more likely that an intimate, or collaborative peer friendship would ensue in which mentoring would tend to be minimal. In Levinson's definition the mentor facilitates life transitions between the ages of 20 and 40 by allowing the mentee to be a 'novice or apprentice to a more advanced, expert and authoritative adult'. Mentors exemplify the qualities that the mentees wish to attain and their values, virtues and accomplishments are eventually internalised by the mentees. Levinson's work has been criticised on several grounds though primarily for the following reasons:

◆ Gender bias – the case studies were all male.
◆ Although Levinson identified the need for a mentor as being common to all men, he did not specify how many of his subjects had mentors which means that a valid evaluation of the role is not possible from his work.
◆ Levinson's suggestion that mentors are characteristically 8–15 years older than their mentees has been criticised on the grounds that it might be more appropriate to consider the quality and experience of the mentor rather than this arbitrary age criterion.

Despite this criticism, however, Levinson's vivid and detailed description of the mentoring relationship has helped to stimulate the imagination of others.

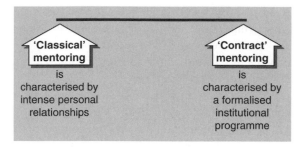

Fig 8.2 The mentoring continuum

Early thinking about mentoring drew heavily on the special mythical qualities of the relationship. The claimed advantages of mentoring led to high expectations of the process which in turn led to developments in training and education programmes intended to incorporate these advantages.

These developments were in line with Clutterbuck's (1985) view that the origins of mentoring are to be found in the concept of apprenticeship. In this sense a mentor becomes involved in a relationship which is initiated, sometimes formally, by an organisation in order to achieve results similar to those of the classical relationship, as part of a structured staff development programme. Managers of staff development programmes began to analyse the functions of the classical relationship so that these could be incorporated into structured training. This led to an emphasis on mentoring as a skills hierarchy with, in some cases, an emphasis on specific outcomes.

The distinction between this instrumental form of mentoring and the more classical notions of the concept (East 1987) is particularly pertinent in nurse education. For Morton-Cooper and Palmer (1993) the notion of mentoring in nurse education as being merely support for tasks linked to professional and vocational qualification would fall into the category of 'pseudo or quasi-mentoring' because the focus is only on getting the qualifications, more akin to support provided by personal tutors. 'True mentoring' of a classical nature is reserved for the holistic support for the individual in the development of a new and complex professional role (see Fig. 8.2).

THE CONCEPTUAL BASES FOR MENTORING

Although there has been little systematic research into the conceptual bases for mentoring there is a considerable amount of published material on the subject. Gray and Gray (1986) and Noller and Frey (1983) provide bibliographies of studies of mentoring in academic settings, adult development programmes, career and business management, education, leadership training, medicine, nursing, psychotherapy and general supervisory/training programmes.

The concepts associated with mentoring are embedded within several theories of human learning and development. Thomas et al (1982) refer to three such theories in their examination of the conceptual base of mentoring:

◆ Life-span development – Erik Erikson.
◆ Stages of intellectual and ethical development – William Perry.
◆ Social learning theory – Albert Bandura.

Life-span development

Erikson's (1969) model of life-span development describes a series of eight stages from birth to old age. Each stage has a 'psychosocial crisis' associated with it as shown in Table 8.2.

Erikson used this term to emphasise that the tasks to be completed are both psychological (in relation to the self) and social (in relation to others) and that there are important developmental issues to be resolved. The stages are age-linked but should not be construed as a series of steps leading to an 'achievement' within a given stage because each stage depends on the previous stages and affects the ones that follow. The outcome of each stage is dependent on the balance between an individual's positive and negative experiences and this tension remains throughout life.

The seventh stage (mid-adulthood) is the stage of most relevance for mentors. The central task of this stage, generativity versus stagnation, is

Table 8.2 Implications of Erikson's eight life stages (adapted from Erikson 1985)

Stage	Age (approx)	Task	Favourable outcome	Unfavourable outcome	Lasting accomplishment of successful outcome
1	Infancy (0–1 year)	Basic trust v. mistrust	Feelings of being wanted and loved and cared for. A sense of stability and order in experience – the result of physical and emotional 'mothering'.	Life is chaotic and unconnected. Child likely to be psychologically and possibly physically disabled. Higher infant mortality than usual. Retardation, possibly autism.	Drive and hope
2	Toddler (1–3 years)	Autonomy v. shame and doubt	Learns to stand on own two feet. Feeds self and begins to control bodily functions and use language to meet basic needs. Learns to say and accept 'no' as well as 'yes'. Begins to learn rules of society.	Lack of autonomy, passive dependence on others. Unable to assert own will, resulting in over-obedience. Paradoxically, is unable to accept 'no' and so results in constantly rebellious personality, perhaps delinquency.	Self-control and will power
3	Pre-school (about 4–5 years)	Initiative v. guilt	Has developed memory, can go and come back, both in place and time. Starts to learn adult gender roles. More loving, cooperative, secure in family. Good chance of becoming able to make moral choices.	Always wants to be 'in control'. Sense of competition drives individual to be over-competitive. May be always outside the law.	Direction and purpose
4	School (about 6–12 years)	Industry v. inferiority	Learns the basic skills of society – the 'how to's, the 'three Rs'. Learns to feel worthy and competent.	If person fails to learn industry, begins to feel inferior compared with others. If over-learns industry, may become too task-oriented and over-conform to society.	Method and competence

(Continued)

Table 8.2 (Continued)

Stage	Age (approx)	Task	Favourable outcome	Unfavourable outcome	Lasting accomplishment of successful outcome
5	Adolescence (age 12 to late teens or early adulthood)	Identity v. role confusion	Sexual maturation and sexual identity. Ponders question 'Who am I?' as distinct from family. Develops social friendships. Tends to reject and be in conflict with family. Begins to discover role in life.	May not achieve an identity separate from family. May not become socially adult or sexually stable.	Devotion and fidelity
6	Early adulthood	Intimacy v. isolation	Learns to share passions, interests, problems with another individual. Also relates to others at work, in community, as well as in family. Achieves stability.	Inability to be intimate with others. Becomes fixated at adolescent level, preoccupied with sensation-seeking and self-pleasure. Avoids responsibility and lacks stability.	Affiliation and love
7	Middle adulthood	Generativity v. self-absorption and stagnation	Fosters creativity and growth in others younger than self. Provides leadership, seeks to contribute to community, next generation, world. 'Minds the store'. May be most creative period of life.	Growth limited, remains rooted in past. Becomes 'cog-in-wheel', automated. May experience breakdown of zest for life. Feels life is passing him/her by.	Production and care
8	Old age	Ego integrity v. despair	Recognises and accepts diminishing faculties. Realises and faces own death. Feeling of having lived a 'good enough' life, paving the way for future generations. Dignity of truly 'wise' person.	Reaps bitter fruits of what was sown or not sown earlier. Fears death. An old age of misery, anxiety and despair.	Renunciation and wisdom

---

Box 8.1 Erikson's seventh stage of lifespan development

The generative person is able to foster creativity and growth in others. This may be the most creative period in a person's life, the culmination of a favourable enough outcome of the preceding stages leading to trust, stability, self-esteem, fidelity, competence, the capacity to work and have concern for others. From this solid foundation the generative person can provide leadership and contribute to the community, the next generation and the world at large.

In contrast, the opposite of generativity is self-absorption and stagnation. If preceding stages have resulted in a person feeling powerless, directionless, rootless and inferior, the capacity to feel concern for others is stunted.

Box 8.2 A negative experience of mentoring

Annie is a very highly qualified and experienced nurse tutor. She is the mentor to Lucy who is in her second year of training. Reflecting on her experience Annie says:

'I don't think I'm overstating to say that my mentee sees me as a minor irritation, a person who has very little more, if any more, expertise than she has. Lucy seems to think "Here's someone who thinks she knows it all. If I want to get this qualification I suppose I've got to tolerate her and be civil but I won't go out of my way to draw on what she might be able to offer me because I don't believe she can offer me anything". She is always reluctant to discuss assignment or project material with me although she's quite prepared to use me as a matter of convenience to deliver work for her. We don't have confrontations but I feel I'm there out of sheer forbearance on her part rather than a desire to achieve something together.'

Lucy finds it difficult to share herself with colleagues at work. She tends to keep herself to herself, feeling somewhat overwhelmed by intimate relationships and has problems with authority figures.

Lucy says 'I know vaguely what it means to have a mentor. If I require help I can chat with her. I don't have a great deal of contact with her actually; she's quite marginal. It's not negative, it's bland. I can take it or leave it.'

---

dependent on the favourable outcomes of the preceding developmental tasks which are likely to give a person a basic trust in the world, hope for the future, a sense of confidence and purpose, and a successful pattern of relating to others (see Box 8.1).

The strengths of the generative person are 'production and care' so these represent core qualities for mentoring construed from Erikson's perspective. Thomas et al refer to the generative person as 'the perfect mentor' and Merriam (1983) claims that 'mentoring is one manifestation of this mid-life task'.

To be able to relate to and use a mentor effectively requires that the mentee is sufficiently mature emotionally to be able to receive support without feeling crushed or overwhelmed by the difference in status and experience. This requires that the mentee has already established an adequate sense of identity and the ability to relate effectively to others, i.e. to have a positive outcome from earlier tasks in stages 5 and 6. See Boxes 8.2 and 8.3 for a description of negative and positive experiences in mentoring.

Intellectual and ethical development

Perry (1981) is concerned to plot the normal expected change in individuals' intellectual and ethical development. In common with other stage theories, Perry's is hierarchical, though the time taken to pass through the stages will vary from individual to individual and the passage may stop or go into reverse, especially if external conditions become too threatening or overwhelming. The nine

Box 8.3 A positive mentoring experience

Edwina is just two years from retirement after a successful career as a nurse practitioner. Ben is a nurse coming towards the end of his training.

Edwina says: 'You see a light at the end of the tunnel and it says retirement above the door and you're just pulling up the ladder to coast home when somebody like Ben comes along. I realise now I am a nurse to the day I retire. There's a lot for me to learn still and my patients benefit even though they never see Ben. I feel basically I am a support unit to the course but one step away from the course so Ben can come to me and explain what his basic problem is with less embarrassment than if he went to one of his tutors. Ben sometimes thinks his questions are stupid questions and they're not – they're very important questions. It reminds me, although I'm very experienced now, of the worries I had when I was a student. It's empathy really.'

Ben says: 'She provides me with a stabilising influence. I like her and I trust her. I feel she can hold a confidence and I have confidence in her. I can lean on her. I was afraid I would reveal too much of myself and she would get fed up with me. I think she's had a difficult role with me because I've been like a barrel of dynamite at times. She's actually handled it very well because she's let *me* work through it. She's got personal qualities in that she leads rather than drives and has this ability to go right to the heart of the matter. As a result when I'm floundering along … I suppose when we're floundering we're all embarrassed but I know she will be able to headline it, just little bits of help, just enough to lift me and carry me through. So I'm very happy with my mentor and I'm very aware of what it must feel like to be handling someone like me. I'm grateful to her. I don't know what else to say except to repeat that I'm grateful.'

positions of Perry's scheme are grouped into four categories (see Fig. 8.3).

The mentor's role begins functioning at position 9 when the mentoring relationship offered is likely to be characterised by independence, flexibility, openness and the ideal combination of support and challenge. The novice in any situation, especially nursing, is likely to be operating at an earlier stage and so can potentially be aided in development by a mentor who 'knows the ropes' and has been through the earlier stages. How often the newcomer wants to know the 'right' way of doing something and, how difficult to realise that there may not be a 'right' way but rather a range of options from which the newcomer must choose.

Social learning theory

Bandura's social learning theory is used to clarify an important aspect of mentoring, i.e. modelling. If the mentor is perceived as a person worthy of emulation, the mentee is likely to imitate the mentor's behaviour, values and attitudes. Such imitation, or modelling, is likely to result from the whole integrated behaviour and actions of the mentor rather than just his words. The mentor might act as a model for the acquisition of complex social and interpersonal skills or, in a situation in which mistakes could be costly and dangerous, a model of safe, confident, clinical behaviour.

In Bandura's definition of modelling, imitation is seen as more than merely copying behaviour and is divided into three categories (see Fig. 8.4).

It is important to note again that this social learning theory is based on operant conditioning (see Chapter 2) and is concerned with reinforcement and imitation principally in relation to behaviour control and modification.

Zey (1984) warns that to call the mentoring relationship role-modelling is to understate the power of the interaction. Referring to the process as 'role participation', a most potent form of learning, Zey claims that this is as different from role-modelling as on-the-job training is from textbook learning. The mentee is not a passive observer but an active participant in the learning process, integrating observational learning into previous learning.

The common theme that runs throughout each of these three theories is that a healthy mentoring

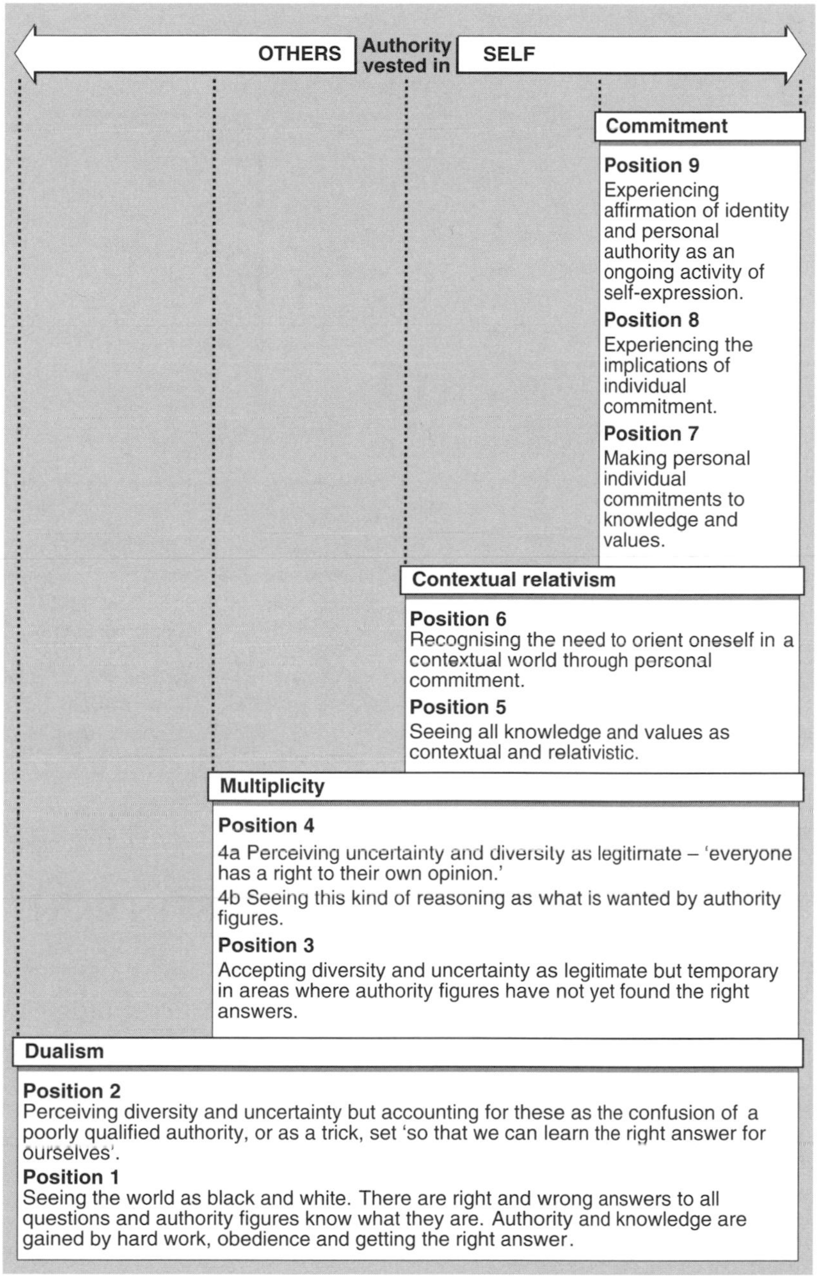

OTHERS | Authority vested in | SELF

Commitment

Position 9
Experiencing affirmation of identity and personal authority as an ongoing activity of self-expression.

Position 8
Experiencing the implications of individual commitment.

Position 7
Making personal individual commitments to knowledge and values.

Contextual relativism

Position 6
Recognising the need to orient oneself in a contextual world through personal commitment.

Position 5
Seeing all knowledge and values as contextual and relativistic.

Multiplicity

Position 4
4a Perceiving uncertainty and diversity as legitimate – 'everyone has a right to their own opinion.'
4b Seeing this kind of reasoning as what is wanted by authority figures.

Position 3
Accepting diversity and uncertainty as legitimate but temporary in areas where authority figures have not yet found the right answers.

Dualism

Position 2
Perceiving diversity and uncertainty but accounting for these as the confusion of a poorly qualified authority, or as a trick, set 'so that we can learn the right answer for ourselves'.

Position 1
Seeing the world as black and white. There are right and wrong answers to all questions and authority figures know what they are. Authority and knowledge are gained by hard work, obedience and getting the right answer.

Fig 8.3 Perry's four stages of intellectual and ethical development

relationship is one where both mentor and mentee have a trusting attitude towards each other. The mentor is able to share ideas and opinions from a clearly articulated value framework, without imposing those ideas and opinions on the mentee. Generative people have the capacity for industry and competence and the ability and desire to foster these strengths in others.

1. OBSERVATIONAL LEARNING

Modelling by imitating any form of behaviour desired by the imitator.

Models might be:

a. **An actual person**
   – peer, colleague, friend.
b. **A symbolic model**
   – fictional character, religious, mythical or legendary figure.
c. **An exemplary model**
   – parent, teacher, boss.

For example :

(a) Su-Lin wants to be as good a nurse as her colleague, Amy, whom she has worked alongside on her initial placement.

(b) Carlos has always found TV hospital dramas compulsive viewing. Now he wants to be a nurse just like his favourite character in a current serial.

(c) Both of David's parents have worked in medical settings and his ambition is to follow their example.

2. INHIBITORY/DISINHIBITORY EFFECTS

Imitation of deviant behaviour may have:

a. **An inhibitory effect**
   – deviant behaviour is seen to be punished and therefore inhibited in the observer.
b. **A disinhibitory effect**
   – deviant behaviour is seen not to be punished and is therefore imitated.

For example:

(a) Lottie observes her friend Irene being disciplined for her continual lateness for work. She makes her own decision to be punctual because she cannot bear the thought of being told off which for her would feel like a humiliation.

(b) Although Mark knows that he should respect confidential information about patients he has observed other staff leaving notes around the ward and that they don't get into trouble. This leads Mark to treat the patients' personal information carelessly and without respect.

Fig 8.4 Bandura's three categories of learning by observation and imitation

3. ELICITING EFFECT

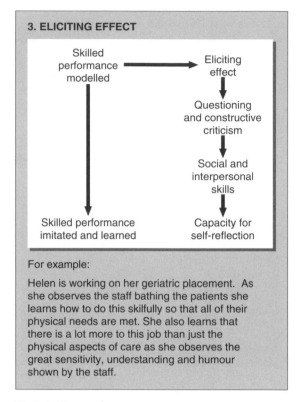

For example:

Helen is working on her geriatric placement. As she observes the staff bathing the patients she learns how to do this skilfully so that all of their physical needs are met. She also learns that there is a lot more to this job than just the physical aspects of care as she observes the great sensitivity, understanding and humour shown by the staff.

Fig 8.4 (*Continued*)

MENTORING IN CONTEXT

Mentoring is a complex and dynamic process and can be implemented in a variety of ways, embracing both classical and instrumental mentoring. This section examines mentoring in the context of large organisations, education and nursing.

Mentoring in organisations

In an organisational setting mentoring may take place within contractual relationships, which are initiated formally by the organisation in order to maintain its cohesion and stability. Within this setting mentoring is implemented as part of a programme of organisational or career development rather than personal adult development, although these are not mutually exclusive.

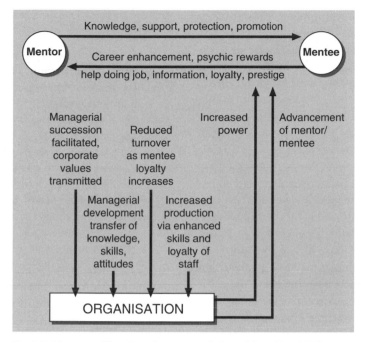

Fig 8.5 The mutual benefits of mentoring (adapted from Zey 1984)

Large firms such as Shell, ICI, the Institute of Chartered Accountants, Local Authorities, NHS Trusts, Primary Care Trusts and Strategic Health Authorities use mentoring as part of their management strategies. Mentoring may be formalised in order to benefit the company or institution or it might focus on new entrants and/or 'high flyers'. There are potential disadvantages in focusing mentoring programmes on a particular group, for example graduates, in that staff excluded from the mentoring programme may feel devalued, disadvantaged and demotivated in comparison.

The concept of mentoring in an organisational setting tends to involve what Zey has described as the 'mutual benefits model' in which the instrumental relationship concerned with the career development of the mentee is expanded to include possible benefits for the mentor, the mentee and the organisation as shown in Figure 8.5.

Problems in the mentoring relationship may arise between the mentor and mentee or between the mentoring pair and the organisation. Any difficulties within the mentor/mentee relationship may stem from poor communication, leading to a mismatch of perceptions, from a failure to communicate needs and goals or from over-dependence. Problems arising between the mentoring pair and the organisation often include a failure on the mentor's part to assess the political environment accurately or an inability to control the political environment. Zey refers to the 'black halo' effect of a politically weak mentor 'contaminating' the mentee.

Whilst recognising mentoring as powerful in human resource development, mentoring should not be the only form of career development within an organisation. A variety of staff development and training opportunities is needed to avoid the dangers of elitism and consequent resentment and to avoid confusion caused by applying the term mentoring to induction programmes or specific short-term tasks.

Mentoring in education

Mentoring programmes are used in a wide variety of educational settings, for example in programmes for gifted children; initial and in-service teacher training and staff development programmes; undergraduate and faculty programmes; small business advice, cooperatives, adult and community programmes and in nurse education which is covered in more detail below. The aims of these programmes include the fostering of independent, self-managed learning; support for open learning projects; and the provision of learning experiences not possible in the classroom or lecture theatre.

Egan (1986) reports on North American State programmes which use 'master-teachers' as a source of support, advice and inspiration for new teachers. Referring to the difficulties during the first 3 years of teaching, Egan asks whether mentors could ease the transition from student to novice teacher to professional teacher. Teaching can be a 'professional desert' for new staff, with communication made difficult by the isolation of classroom experiences and a fear of discussing problems or asking too many questions because of the risk of appearing incompetent.

Teachers may need different types of mentoring at different points in their careers. The new teacher needs to deal with survival in the classroom; the more experienced teacher may need discussion on the complex issues of education. Neil (1986) supports this progression of changing needs, referring to the teacher in the first year of teaching as being self-oriented; in the second and third years of teaching as being teacher-oriented; and in the fourth year as being pupil-centred. Mentoring programmes in education could form the basis of collaborative in-service training, and would be valuable for supportive work including mutual planning; demonstration of teaching techniques; structured feedback; developing strengths and skills and allowing risk-taking in a safe environment.

Egan refers to the many roles that mentors play in in-service training and claims that mentees speak glowingly about the opportunity to observe their mentors teaching. This is viewed as real opportunity to see theory being put into practice (see Box 8.4).

This form of role-modelling enables new teachers to observe some features of teaching that are difficult to learn in any other way. For example,

---

Box 8.4 A teaching observation

'In lots of ways he was a classic person for me to have as a mentor because I've got a lot of respect for his track record. He's obviously been teaching a long time and watching him teach was quite an amazing experience. He has terrific humour, he's very approachable. There's a lot of laughter with him. He teaches very dry subjects but at the same time he has this ability to relate it to silly everyday events which are actually valid analogies. Being slightly ridiculous it makes the students laugh but at the same time they remember the concepts.'

'student-centredness' and appropriate forms of communication and behaviour in the classroom might only be learned in this way.

Mentoring in nursing

The role of the mentor in nursing has been examined as part of the UKCC-initiated reforms which have had a profound effect on nursing and nurse education. The core studies component of Making a Difference comprises an ever-increasing body of knowledge and, whilst this is important, there are aspects of nursing which require more than knowledge alone. For example, one has only to look at Clause 4 of the Nursing and Midwifery Councils Code of Professional Conduct which states that 'you (the nurse) are expected to work co-operatively within the teams and to respect the skills, expertise and contributions of your colleagues.'

The interpretation and application of this clause, and of the whole Code, can only be developed in the context of a collaborative and cooperative relationship with more experienced colleagues. The dynamic interplay of skills, knowledge, understanding, professional attitudes and values is embedded in the concept of the reflective practitioner.

On current courses all students have some form of mentorship throughout the clinical practice elements of their course and there is now a common acceptance that this mentoring should be the responsibility of practitioners in the field rather than of nurse tutors. So what is the evidence that, in practice, there are benefits to students from such mentors and what are the characteristics of mentors that are helpful?

Generally students recognise that having a mentor is beneficial and most accounts recall positive aspects of the mentor/mentee alliance. Reports from students usually highlight a mentor's interpersonal skills, such as being approachable and supportive. Also being keen and enthusiastic about their job, yet realistic in their expectations, gives students positive role models and hope for their future. When students feel supported and comfortable in a clinical area they learn more effectively, showing, not surprisingly, that their learning is less to do with direct transference of knowledge than with the nature of the relationship between mentor and student, in line with what was said earlier (Andrews & Wallis 1999).

Gray and Smith (2000) did a longitudinal study to investigate changes in the students' perspective of their mentor over time, first, prior to the first placement experience and then, after four practice placements. At the start the mentor was seen as playing a major role and students realised how vital their mentor would be to their learning.

Student: 'It makes me feel a lot better actually ... while I am trying to find my feet I am glad there is somebody in particular to guide me. I don't think I will feel as bad going up to my mentor and saying "Look I don't know how to do something, can you show me how it's done or explain this to me". I don't think I would feel as easy going up to any of the other staff nurses because I think that they have enough on their plate so I shouldn't be bothering them. Whereas I know that is what my mentor is there for.'

After four placements, having a mentor remains an important issue but there is a realisation that a mentor has competing priorities and is not there exclusively for the individual student.

Student: 'I think as a student you are very aware of how your mentors are pulled and pushed in so many directions and it is difficult to actually sit down in a way and get the time to spend together .... On your first placement you believe you are the most important thing apart from the patients on the ward for your mentor but you certainly soon realise, perhaps within the space of an hour(!), that you are one of the many pressing priorities'.

In the last 18 months of their course the students commented on the gradual distancing of themselves from their mentor, this movement being related to their growing self-confidence and their familiarity with ward routines. The mentor's main roles then move towards teaching and giving constructive criticism, seen as crucial. Students felt strongly that without a good mentor their learning experience would suffer because it is the mentor who would, or would not, let students see and do things, allow or refuse independence and initiative, encouraging personal development from observation to participation.

At the end of their course, as well as contemplating their future role as staff nurses, students thought about how they would perform themselves as future mentors, based on their experience of being mentees. Box 8.5 gives a list of the qualities of a good mentor that they aspired to.

In summary all this suggests that effective mentoring in nursing relies on good training and communication between all parties involved. Andrews and Wallis (1999) conclude their literature review by saying:

'If mentorship schemes are to be effective there is a need for stronger communication links between mentors, practitioner teams and those responsible for nurse education. Nurse teachers have an ongoing responsibility for quality monitoring aspects for their courses and for mentoring practitioners undertaking a mentoring role.'

Research and mentoring

Although until recently American experiences are often quoted as the source of mentoring initiatives in Great Britain, questions about their effectiveness

Box 8.5 Students' perceptions of a good mentor (from Gray & Smith 2000)

◆ Support the student rather than breathe down their neck.

◆ Encourage and allow involvement and participation in patient care rather than just observation.

◆ Show confidence in the student's abilities and trust them to do things unsupervised.

◆ Form a relaxed relationship with their student.

◆ Take time every day to let the student do or observe something and not assume that because they were in a certain team they would have already seen or performed it.

◆ Regardless of the student's stage, have an initial discussion, preferably on the first day, to determine what the student's present abilities are and their intended learning outcomes for the placement.

◆ Ascertain what the student required as an individual to meet the desired learning outcomes.

◆ Clarify ground on both sides and discuss the opportunities available to meet desired learning outcomes.

◆ Remember the student if there was anything interesting happening on the ward.

◆ Allow the student some independence by giving more guidance at the beginning of the placement. They would stand back and let the student show initiative and self-motivation.

◆ Make arrangements with other members of staff to 'look out for them' if they were going to be off duty when the student was on duty rather than have the student feel abandoned.

◆ Think carefully about the duty rota in terms of arranging shifts to allow student and mentor to work together at some point each week.

are also asked in the United States. Surveying the American scene, Hagerty (1986) provides a critical analysis of mentoring literature and examines the concept and theory, basic assumptions, related research, and the resulting generalisations and implications. Cautious and sceptical about some of the more florid claims made in support of mentoring from earlier studies, Hagerty points out that these assertions have been laid on weak foundations. Some studies confused their definition of mentor by including it in a range of supportive roles; others did not include any definition at all.

The samples used for research on mentoring have been small, selective, atypical and nonrandom. There has been little use of control groups and research methods have tended to be descriptive, retrospective and anecdotal. Thus, conclusions and implications based on existing research are likely to be unsupported and inappropriate. Hagerty further claims that research studies have too often been merely a description of activities and there has been confusion about whether it is the person or the process, the purposes or the activities which are being described.

There have been many assumptions made about mentoring and although these are sometimes unexamined they are often presented as facts. Common assumptions include the belief that having a mentor is a requisite for success and that is why women do not succeed; that the only success that counts is upward mobility through the organisational hierarchy; and that mentoring is the same across all work settings.

In Britain, concerns have been expressed about the absence of a clear definition of mentoring (Armitage & Burnard 1991, Morle 1990). These authors go on to introduce the idea of 'preceptorship' – an individual teaching/learning method in which students are assigned to 'preceptors' who act as clinical role models – as an alternative for helping to bridge the theory/practice gap. Anforth (1992) reviews these arguments in her own clarification of the mentoring role and concludes that it should be retained in addition to the roles of preceptor, facilitator and assessor.

Assessment and mentoring

Mentoring programmes in nurse education highlight perhaps more sharply than in other settings the question of whether the role of mentor should include an assessment function. Can a mentor also act as assessor when he is perhaps working with, and helping, students who may be fearful of those with power? In this situation adult students might mask their anxieties and uncertainties with bravado if they fear that expressing uncertainty could affect their assessments.

Anforth, together with Morton-Cooper and Palmer, stresses the benefits of developing rapport between mentor and mentee, ideally in a continuous relationship which lasts throughout the training period, and the need for this to be separated from assessment procedures. This approach is much disputed. For example, describing the Torbay mentoring scheme, Morris et al (1988) include the assessment role as one of four main mentoring roles: role model/facilitator/supervisor/assessor. They see the mentor as the 'obvious candidate' to be the student's assessor.

In the Torbay scheme the mentors, all mental health nurses, are given a week's training and are audited on their skills in mentoring. Learners are allocated to mentors on the basis of these audited skills rather than clinical areas. The average time spent in a mentoring relationship is 6 months and the mentor acts as an 'enabler/catalyst'. Morris et al do not advocate an 'inseparable bonding', instead they envisage a tripartite relationship between learner, mentor and tutor.

Potential/transitional space

Even though the nursing profession is constantly being redefined, it still demands certainty in many areas, particularly clinical areas. It may be difficult to incorporate models of training that allow for individual interpretation of an abstract, some would say slippery and elusive, concept such as mentoring. Some staff will need clarity imposed from the outside, others will feel comfortable in

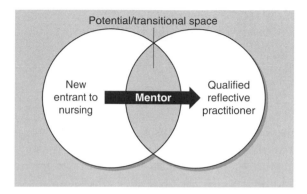

Fig 8.6 The area of potential/transitional space

determining their own clarity. If nursing is claiming the title of profession then staff must be prepared for a role which incorporates and encourages autonomy.

The changes in nurse education herald a period of transition. Institutions must manage transitions efficiently if they are to survive. Learning that takes place during such periods might be compared with Winnicott's (1982) ideas on transitional phenomena, which are concentrated in the space between inner and outer experiences.

It is in this 'potential space' that children learn to play and, if they are fortunate, continue to do so throughout their lives in active, exploratory learning which enables them to create their own understanding and insight. This idea lies at the heart of student-centred learning. Mentoring takes place within the potential space between two people. The result is the outcome of what they are able to create together (see Fig. 8.6).

Mentoring programmes need to encompass not only the development of competent clinical nurses but also the development of an individual's ability to become self-directing and thoughtful – the reflective practitioner.

SO WHAT IS A MENTOR?

The research into the conceptual bases for mentoring and its application in organisational, educational and nursing settings reveals the complexity of the role of a mentor. Cross (1976) reviewed the skill classifications in the US Dictionary of Occupational titles and found that mentoring was listed as the most complex role in terms of required interpersonal skills.

This complexity has led to a failure by some researchers to conceptualise the role. There has also been a variety of uses of the word mentor so that the definition varies from study to study. Mentoring is too complex for an adequate description through the use of a single procedure.

Given this complexity it is not surprising that research into the application of mentoring in organisational, educational and nursing settings has tended to break the concept down into its functional components. In nursing this has led to confusion about the nature of mentoring and the similarities and differences between this and preceptorship and tutoring.

It may be worth distinguishing between the need to get the 'right' definition and the need to have a 'clear' definition. The classical interpretation of the role leads us into metaphor and thence into personal interpretation. The desire for a clear definition of the role may indicate difficulty in coping with the tension of a complex, interpersonal role rooted in subjective experience. This tension may be resolved by resorting to an operational definition and being prescriptive about what a mentor is expected to do. There will always be differences in personal interpretation of the role: sometimes a nurse mentor will be a classical mentor; sometimes an instrumental mentor.

The development of appropriate interpersonal skills is highly important to the success of a mentoring relationship characterised by an interactional dialogue, shared problem solving and mutual exploration. These skills have a broad overlap with the skills of counselling described in Chapter 7.

If mentoring is construed as a bridging process between theory and practice it can serve several levels of activity, spanning not only induction and initial training but also continuing professional development for practitioners and managers. The stronger the bridge, the more confident the mentoring pair and the more frequent the journeys across the bridge, backwards and forwards, from not knowing to knowing, from not understanding to understanding, in an on-going process until eventually theory becomes integrated into practice. As a result of being mentored it is hoped that the mentee will become an autonomous professional who is self-reflective and self-directing.

Mentoring is not something that is given or done to others, it is about the relationships between people. What distinguishes fine mentors is their capacity and willingness to care. They know that they exist as mentors only because they are part of a relationship.

REFERENCES

Andrews M, Wallis M 1999 Mentoring in nursing: a literature review. Journal of Advanved Nursing 29(1): 201–207

Anforth P 1992 Mentors, not assessors. Nurse Education 12: 299–302

Armitage P, Burnard P 1991 Mentors or preceptors? Narrowing the theory practice gap. Nurse Education Today 11: 223–229

Bandura A 1977 Social learning theory. Englewood Cliffs, Prentice Hall, New Jersey

Bandura A, Walters RH 1963 Social learning and personality development. Holt, Rinehart & Winston, New York

Campbell-Holder N 1986 Do nurses need mentors? Image 183: 110–113

Clutterbuck D 1985 Everybody needs a mentor: how to foster talent within the organisation. IPM, London

Cross KP 1976 Accent on learning, improving instruction and re-shaping the curriculum. Jossey Bass, San Francisco

Daloz LA 1986 Effective teaching and mentoring: realising the transformational power of adult learning experiences. Jossey-Bass, San Francisco

East PI 1987 The mentoring relationship. Unpublished MA thesis, University of Loughborough

Egan JB 1986 Characteristics of classroom teachers mentor–protege relationships. In: Gray W, Gray MM (eds) Mentoring: an aid to excellence, Vol. I, International Association for Mentoring, Vancouver, Canada

Erikson E 1969 Childhood and society, 2nd edn. Norton, New York

Gray M, Smith L 2000 The qualities of an effective mentor from the student nurse's perspective: findings from a longitudinal qualitative study. Journal of Advanced Nursing 32(6): 1542–1549

Gray WA, Gray MM 1986 A comprehensive annotated bibliography of important references. International Association for Mentoring, Vancouver, Canada

Gray WA, Gray MM 1986 Mentoring: aid to excellence. Proceedings of the 1st International Conference on Mentoring, vols I and II. International Association for Mentoring, Vancouver, Canada

Hagerty B 1986 A second look at mentors. Nursing Outlook 34(1): 16–24

Kegan R 1982 The evolving self. London, Harvard University Press

Levinson D 1978 The seasons of a man's life. Alfred Knopf, New York

Merriam SS 1983 Mentors and proteges: A critical review of the literature. Adult Education Quarterly Spring: 161–173

Morle KM 1990 Mentorship   is it a case of the emperor's new clothes or a rose by any other name? Nurse Education Today 10(1): 66–69

Morris N, John G, Keen T 1988 Mentors: learning the ropes. Nursing Times 84(46): 24–27

Morton-Cooper A, Palmer A 1993 Mentoring and preceptorship. Blackwell Scientific, Oxford

Neil R 1986 Current models and approaches to in-service teacher education. British Journal of In-service Education 12(2): 58–67

Noller RB, Frey B 1983 Mentoring: an annotated bibliography. Brearly Ltd, New York

Perry WG 1981 Cognitive and ethical growth: the making of meaning. In: Chickering AE (ed) 1981 The modern American college. Jossey-Bass, San Francisco

Rowntree D 1981 A dictionary of education. Harper & Row, London

Thomas R, Murrell PH, Chickering AW 1982 Theoretical bases and feasibility issues for mentoring and developmental transcripts. In: Brown RD, De Coster DA (eds) 1982 Mentoring transcript systems for promoting student growth. New directions for student services, No 19. Jossey Bass, San Francisco

Winnicott DW 1982 The maturational processes and the facilitating environment: studies in the theory of emotional development. The Hogarth Press Ltd and the Institute of Psycho-Analysis, London

Zey MG 1984 The mentor connection. Dow Jones Irwin, Illinois

FURTHER READING

Baker S 1990 The key to nurse education. Nursing Standard 4: 39–43

Brown RD, De Coster DA (eds) 1982 Mentoring transcript systems for promoting student growth. In: New directions for student services No 19. Jossey Bass, San Francisco

Butterworth T, Faugier J 1992 Clinical supervision and mentorship in nursing. Chapman & Hall, London

Donovan J 1990 The concept and role of mentor. Nurse Education Today 10(4): 294–298

Knowles M 1973 The adult learner: a neglected species. Gulf Publishing Company, Houston

Knowles M 1986 Using learning contracts. Jossey-Bass, San Francisco

Kram EK 1988 Mentoring at work: developmental relationships in organisational life. University Press of America, Lanham, USA

Monaghan J, Lunt N 1992 Mentoring: person process practice and problems. British Journal of Educational Studies No 3

Rogers CR 1951 Client centred therapy. Houghton, Boston

Rogers CR 1969 Freedom to learn. Merrill, Columbus, Ohio

Rogers CR 1974 On becoming a person. Constable, London

Rothera M, Howkins S, Hendry J et al 1991 The role of subject mentor in further education. British Journal of In-service Education 17(2): 126–137

Speizer JJ 1981 Role models, mentors and sponsors: The elusive concepts in signs. Journal of Women in Culture and Society 6(4): 1981

Talbert EG, Phelps MS 1986 Technical skills of mentoring: a training module for teacher mentors. A paper presented to the 1st International Conference on Mentoring, 24th July 1986. Vancouver, Canada

Tough A 1979 The adult's learning projects, 2nd edn. Ontario Institute for Studies in Education, Toronto

Wrightsman LS 1981 Research methodologies for assessing mentoring. A paper presented to the Annual meeting of the American Psychological Association, Los Angeles, August 1981. In: Gray W, Gray MM (eds) A comprehensive annotated bibliography of important references. International Association for Mentoring, Vancouver, Canada

9

Making the most of clinical supervision

Andy Betts

INTRODUCTION

From a communication perspective, the clinical supervisory relationship shares many of the characteristics and skills of the counselling relationship (see Chapter 7). To be effective they both require a relationship that is established on certain core conditions or values, interpersonal skills that are predominantly facilitative and an unambiguous focus on the experiences of one party. There are two main aspects that discriminate counselling and clinical supervision. First, clinical supervision focuses exclusively on work-related issues, unlike counselling which has no such restriction. Second, that the clinical supervisor has a responsibility not only to the supervisee, but also to a third party, namely the patient or client who receives care from the supervisee.

This chapter highlights aspects of clinical supervision with a particular focus on the communication processes and interpersonal skills that underpin effective practice.

DEFINING CLINICAL SUPERVISION

In the United Kingdom (UK) clinical supervision has been prominent on the nursing agenda for almost ten years since it was highlighted in the Report of the Chief Nursing Officer (Department of Health 1993). This decade of activity has been characterised by a preoccupation with defining what clinical supervision actually is and, by implication, what it is not. The reasons for this distraction are complex and beyond the remit of this chapter, but the consequent confusion, resistance and mistrust have resulted in a patchy uptake of clinical supervision practice in nursing in the UK and a missed opportunity to integrate clinical supervision into everyday practice. For example, Hanson and Betts (1998) surveyed 162 nurses who had attended a course to prepare them for clinical supervision and found that only 38 were engaged in regular clinical supervision activity 12 months following the completion of the course.

As mentioned, the UK nursing literature is replete with definitions of clinical supervision (e.g. Barber & Norman 1987, Bond & Holland 1998, Butterworth & Faugier 1992, Department of Health 1993, Dexter & Wash 1995, Faugier 1994, Kohner 1994, Platt-Koch 1986, UKCC 1996, to name but a few). Each of these definitions emphasises the particular elements that the respective authors regard as most significant. The fact that it is difficult to pick an argument with any of them suggests that the term 'clinical supervision' encompasses many ideas and functions. Perhaps this is not surprising when seen in the context of the diversity of nursing practice.

At the risk of adding a further definition, it is possible to pick out essential elements from these definitions, namely, reflection, structure, work focus and an attentive third party. It is the context of the nursing speciality and environment that will determine the specific translation of these elements into clinical supervision activity.

There is also a general consensus that clinical supervision is a learning dialogue, for example the King's Fund (Kohner 1994) states that it is 'A formal arrangement that allows nurses, midwives and health visitors to discuss their work with another experienced professional … (clinical supervision) involves reflecting on practice in order to learn from experience and improve competence.' (Kohner 1994).

Clinical supervision is essentially a mechanism for reflection and can occur in pairs or groups. The communication skills required of the clinical supervisor are predominantly facilitative and are aimed at enabling the supervisee to explore, clarify and increase options. As clinical supervision becomes better established within the culture of nursing, the communication skills required of clinical supervisors and supervisees will be seen increasingly as important elements of the nurse's role (Activity 9.1).

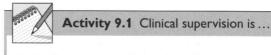

Activity 9.1 Clinical supervision is …

Critically review the definitions of clinical supervision cited and select the one that best fits your own work setting and personal preference.

'an interpersonal process where a skilled practitioner helps a less skilled or experienced practitioner to achieve professional abilities appropriate to his role. At the same time they are offered counsel and support' (Barber & Norman 1987)

'an exchange between practising professionals to enable the development of professional skills' (Butterworth & Faugier 1992)

'a term used to describe a formal process of professional support and learning which enables individual practitioners to develop knowledge and competence, assume responsibility for their own practice and enhance consumer protection in complex clinical situations.' (Department of Health 1993)

'a formal arrangement that enables nurse, midwives and health visitors to discuss their work regularly with another experienced professional. Clinical supervision involves reflecting upon practice in order to learn from experience and improve competence.' (Kohner 1994)

'Clinical supervision brings practitioners and skilled supervisors together to reflect on practice. It aims to identify solutions to problems, improve practice and increase understanding of professional issues.' (UKCC 1996)

'Clinical supervision is regular, protected time for facilitated, in-depth reflection on clinical practice' (Bond & Holland 1998)

POTENTIAL BENEFITS OF CLINICAL SUPERVISION

There is almost universal acceptance within nursing literature that clinical supervision is a good idea. It has to be said that this acceptance is largely based on the beliefs of influential nursing leaders and involves acts of faith rather than hard evidence. The claimed benefits fit within three categories: first, that clinical supervision enhances the quality of care and protection available to patients/clients; second, that clinical supervision is a dialogue that promotes learning (particularly through reflection-on-action and by increasing options); third, that clinical supervision supports the nurse as an individual working in a stressful environment. These three strands have been described by Proctor (1987) as normative, formative and restorative respectively.

The absence of evidence for these claims is unsurprising. For example, the methodological problems involved in ascertaining whether the quality of care received by patient X is enhanced because nurse Y receives regular supervision from supervisor Z are considerable. Despite these complexities White et al (1998) highlight the need for unequivocal evidence for a causal relationship between clinical supervision and improved patient outcomes. At the risk of flying in the face of the current emphasis on evidence-based practice, perhaps common sense should prevail. Professionals working in psychotherapy and counselling universally accept the inherent value of regular supervision on face value, despite the lack of evaluative research. Quality nursing practice requires reflection and sometimes this is better done aloud. Nurses do much of this in staff rooms, offices, tea breaks and nursing stations, and for some this may be sufficient, but the structure and disciplined focus of regular clinical supervision is an additional mechanism worthy of consideration (Activity 9.2).

Perhaps asking the question 'is clinical supervision good for nursing?' is a bit like asking 'is parenting good for a child's development?'. The answer depends on the nature and quality of the

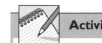

Activity 9.2 Why clinical supervision?

Identify the potential benefits of clinical supervision using the following three categories: benefits to patients/clients; benefits to supervisees; benefits to the organisation.

contact. In this sense the interesting enquiry relates to the process rather than outcomes and the more useful question is not whether the potential benefits of clinical supervision justify the investment, but what specifically makes the difference between effective and ineffective supervision.

The fact that clinical supervision is outside of other formal structures such as management, appraisal, clinical audit and quality assurance monitoring means that it is potentially a more discreet and individualised mechanism. This distinctiveness complements the other more transparent structures as noted by Butterworth and Woods (1998) who recommend that clinical supervision should take place within the overall framework of clinical governance rather than being seen as an activity carried out in isolation.

APPROACHES TO CLINICAL SUPERVISION

There are several types of clinical supervision each with its own particular strengths and limitations. The different types of supervision suit according to people and context. Figure 9.1 illustrates a simple matrix showing the possible types to consider.

One-to-one peer clinical supervision

This approach consists of regular exchanges between two nurses of similar status, with equivalent levels of experience and expertise. It is an opportunity to share similar experiences and compare individual reactions, responses and choices. Usually

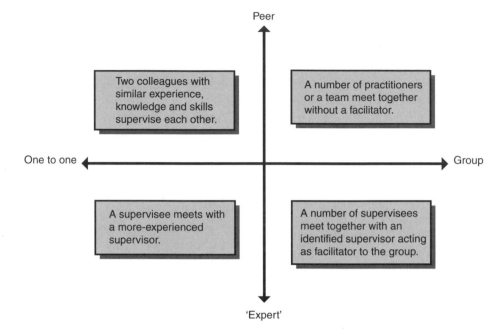

Fig 9.1 Types of clinical supervision

the meetings are reciprocal in the sense that the time is divided equally to reflect on each partner's issues. The advantages of this approach include the mutuality and safety of an equal relationship which may result in a less inhibited dialogue and the sense of universality that derives from the experience of 'being in the same boat'. Disadvantages include the potential for an overcollusive relationship that lacks the structure and challenge required of effective clinical supervision. This lack of structure can result in degeneration into chatting, rather than focused reflection and feedback.

One-to-one 'expert' clinical supervision

The term 'expert' is used advisedly in this context to represent the fact that one party is clearly identified as supervisor and one as supervisee. Usually the supervisor has been selected on the basis of a higher level of experience and possession of the required clinical supervision skills. The main advantage of this approach is that the responsibilities are more clearly demarcated in that the supervisor is not distracted from the central task of 'holding the supervision space'. The entire session focuses on the work experiences of the supervisee, freeing up the supervisor to pay exclusive attention to the content and process of the exchange.

Peer group clinical supervision

Bond and Holland (1998, p. 171) define a supervision group as 'three or more people who come together and interrelate cooperatively with each other towards their common purpose of giving and receiving clinical supervision'. An example of such a group is the peer clinical supervision group. This approach consists of three or more nurses meeting and sharing responsibility for the facilitation of the group. Sometimes teams meet in this way to discuss work. The principle of each member having access to equal time is important and may be more difficult to maintain in the absence of a dedicated facilitator. The risk of the dialogue being dominated by the more verbose members of the group is significant.

The peer group has the advantages noted in peer one-to-one supervision, plus this option may be attractive from a resource point of view, both in terms of the total time away from work, and the scarcity of appropriately trained group clinical supervisors. The other notable advantage of any group supervision is that individual members receive the benefit of multiple contributions, opinions and feedback. Blackford and Street (1998) note the potential for peer group supervision in terms of overcoming frustrations and dilemmas of the job, but caution that the encounters may become hierarchical rather than collaborative.

Facilitated (expert) group clinical supervision

In this case the identified facilitator takes on the responsibility of managing the group structure and process. This liberates the members, enabling them to focus on the content, and makes it less likely that issues such as individual dominators will be allowed to disrupt the sessions. A disadvantage is that the skills required to facilitate such a group and simultaneously respond to the content of what members bring to clinical supervision are considerable. Consequently, it may be difficult to find people with the experience and training required for the role. There are two distinct styles of facilitated group supervision; one consists of the facilitator providing clinical supervision to each group member in turn. In this case the other group members are passive in terms of interacting but active in their involvement as vicarious learners. The second, and arguably more productive style, consists of continuous discussion between group members as each member's issues are introduced in turn. Here the facilitator's role is to facilitate the group interaction and sometimes to sit back and let them get on with it.

When considering which type of clinical supervision fits best for each situation, there are several issues to consider. These include resource issues, level of skills and experience, personal preferences and existing working relationships. From a communication perspective, substantive additional interpersonal skills and understanding are required of a group supervisor in comparison to a one-to-one supervisor. From a resource angle group supervision may appear the appropriate choice but success is dependent on the availability of supervisors who have the necessary facilitative skills and knowledge of group processes required of the role.

The selection of a clinical supervisor will partly depend on the type of clinical supervision.

SETTING UP CLINICAL SUPERVISION

It has been argued that clinical supervision should be contextually determined and consequently, the imposition of any kind of formula is inappropriate; rather what is required is a set of principles. The following suggestions may be worthy of consideration when introducing clinical supervision into nursing.

◆ A general consensus on the function of clinical supervision as complementary but distinct from other quality, managerial and developmental activities.
◆ Organisational support and commitment to individual units.
◆ All staff involved in the planning and implementation to promote ownership.
◆ A contextual evaluation of the strengths and limitations of the different types of clinical supervision, i.e. one-to-one, group, peer, expert.
◆ Supervisors are chosen by supervisees, not allocated.
◆ Supervisors and supervisees are adequately prepared for their roles.
◆ Clinical supervision occurs at all levels of the organisation.
◆ Contracting between parties on structure, respective responsibilities and expectations.
◆ A high prioritisation on the part of both parties (owned not imposed).
◆ Supervisee is responsible for content and supervisor is responsible for the process.

◆ Time and space are protected from intrusion and erosion.
◆ Examines 'good and not so good' practice; supportive yet challenging.
◆ Use of an appropriate, coherent and flexible model of reflection.
◆ Ongoing evaluation is incorporated.

FIRST CONTACT

The first contact between potential supervisor and supervisee requires explicit negotiation (Box 9.1). It is important that both parties discuss their expectations before agreeing to set up a clinical supervision contract. The contract formalises the relationship and distinguishes it from other existing forms of professional support. Each contract will be unique but should cover a number of issues.

Assuming that both parties agree to work together, this first negotiation results in an explicit contract that outlines how the supervision will proceed. This may be written (see Box 9.3) or verbal and will include a summary of the respective responsibilities of both parties. Page and Wosket (1994, p. 67) define a contract as 'an ongoing process which shapes and provides structure and direction to the relationship and the task'. Hawkins and Shohet (2000) propose five key areas that should be covered in the contracting negotiations.

Practicalities

Agreement needs to be reached on the frequency, duration, timing and venue for supervision sessions. Clearly, this will depend on a number of factors, including availability, organisational backing, the demands of the job, existing mechanisms of support and attention timespan. A decision on the frequency of sessions often involves a degree of compromise in nursing contexts. The difference between what is ideal and what is realistic may be influenced by consideration of the implications for colleagues of time away from the work environment or the spare capacity of the supervisor. It is unlikely that clinical supervision will substantively improve things unless

---

Box 9.1 Example of early negotiations

Potential supervisor: 'A good place to start is for you to tell me what you hope to get from clinical supervision.'

Practitioner: 'Well, I have never had clinical supervision before, so I am a bit in the dark … but I have read about it in the nursing journals. I want a safe place where I can talk about my work and get advice. As you know, I work in the Accident and Emergency Department which is sometimes very stressful and demanding. I often go home feeling tense and exhausted and worry about aspects of the job.'

Potential supervisor: 'Yes, I have heard how demanding A & E work can be although I have never worked there myself, apart from a short placement during my training. I agree that for clinical supervision to work well the relationship has to feel "safe". You mentioned advice … my view is that this will not form a large part of what I am able to give you, particularly as I have no recent experience in your specialism. There may be times when I can offer suggestions or alternatives … but more often I will be helping you to make sense of your work experiences, to think about them on a deeper level and encouraging you to come up with alternatives. It may be that supervision could also help you to worry less about your work. What do you think?'

Practitioner: 'At first I thought that it was important that my supervisor was an experienced A & E nurse but I'm not sure that is the most important thing. I have known you for a few years and chose you because of who you are and your experience in supervising other nurses. What you have said so far has not altered this.'

---

it happens at least once a month. The 60-minute session seems to be the optimum for one-to-one supervision although this is often extended for group supervision. Finding a suitable venue that is free from distraction is vital and may prove particularly difficult in hospital settings. These negotiations are not just pragmatic but are symbolic of the level of commitment in ensuring that the clinical supervision 'space' is important to both parties.

Another important practicality is the writing, storage and access to records of clinical supervision. If the supervisor maintains records then it will need to be made explicit what type of records, who has access to them and assurance given that they are securely stored.

Boundaries

The potential for clinical supervision to be confused with either counselling or management is real. Counselling and clinical supervision share similar qualities in terms of the relationship and interpersonal skills. The difference is that supervision is, by definition, work focused, a restriction not shared by counselling. In reality this distinction may become blurred (see Box 9.2). This example illustrates the supervision triad in action. Unlike counselling work the supervisor has a responsibility for a third party, i.e. the client or patient.

Some of the suspicion of clinical supervision within nursing derives from the confusion with hierarchical management functions. Clinical supervision is concerned with empowerment rather than control (Smith 1995). It is important to discuss how these mechanisms are separate. This is partly achieved through clear negotiations on confidentiality and record keeping. The consensus in the literature is that the selection or allocation of one's manager as a supervisor is potentially problematic (Fish and Twinn 1997, Swain 1995) although there are some published examples where this is claimed to work (Kohner 1994), but the potential conflict of 'wearing two hats' has implications for both supervisor and supervisee. It is hard to imagine that the supervisee will not feel some degree of inhibition when disclosing aspects of everyday practice to their supervisor who also happens to be their manager. If the manager is the clinical supervisor then very careful negotiation and regular evaluation are required.

The nature and limits of confidentiality are central to the contracting process, indeed the working

Box 9.2 The boundary of counselling and clinical supervision

James is a community psychiatric nurse who uses his supervision time to discuss his work with a 35-year-old female client whom he is trying to support through a complex grief reaction. Since her father's sudden death 3 years ago she has been depressed and anxious to the extent that she rarely goes out of the house except to spend hours at her father's grave. As James talks about his relationship with the client it becomes apparent to his supervisor that James' own experience of grieving for his mother who died 18 months ago following a long illness is affecting his work with the client.

This example reveals the potential grey area between counselling and clinical supervision. In order to ensure that the client receives the best possible care the supervisor has to pay attention to James' own bereavement. The dilemma is to know where supervision stops and counselling starts. Following some discussion it is agreed by both parties that James will seek support outside of clinical supervision in respect of his own grief (the supervisor is able to suggest somebody who may help with this). This frees the supervisor up to limit attention to James' experience in respect of how it impacts on the client. In other words personal material should only come into the session if it is directly affecting, or being affected by, the work being discussed. This still remains a difficult task and the supervisor makes a mental note to take this to her own supervision session.

alliance is essentially grounded in the spirit of confidentiality. Hawkins and Shohet (2000) point out the mistake made by some new supervisors of offering or implying complete confidentiality, only to find that an unexpected situation compromises this stance. Cutcliffe et al (1998) use six vignettes to illustrate some of the ethical dilemmas that may face clinical supervisors and suggest principles that could inform any contract. These are explicit in the

---

Box 9.3 Example of a clinical supervision contract

We agree to:

◆ Meet each month for one hour at a pre-arranged time and place.

◆ Protect that time and place from interruptions.

◆ Focus on issues selected by ……….. (supervisee) arising from practice.

◆ Review the clinical supervision after six sessions to evaluate objectives.

◆ Maintain a supervision record of contacts and brief notes as an aide-memoir. This record will be kept secure by …………… (supervisor).

As supervisee I agree to:

◆ Prepare for each session by identifying appropriate issues to discuss.

◆ Be open to ideas discussed and review my practice in the light of this.

As supervisor I agree to:

◆ keep all information that is revealed during supervision confidential, except if you reveal any practice that I judge to be unsafe, unethical, negligent or illegal and you are unwilling to go through the appropriate organisational procedures to deal with it yourself.

In these circumstances I will:

i. attempt to convince and support you to deal with the issue through the appropriate channels;

ii. and, if this does not happen, as a last resort reveal the information to the appropriate authorities, informing you of my actions at the time.

◆ Support and challenge you in an attempt to enhance your clinical practice, increase learning and deal with demanding situations.

◆ Not allow any management or assessment functions to be part of our clinical supervision relationship.

◆ Maximise my effectiveness as a clinical supervisor through my own clinical supervision, respecting confidentiality.

Signed _____ (supervisee)

_____ (supervisor)

---

specimen contract (Box 9.3) Nurses are covered by their respective codes of conduct and supervisors should point out their responsibility to the patients or clients receiving care from the supervisees. This involves an awareness of the importance of ethical thinking and debate (Kohner 1996).

Confidentiality in group supervision requires particular attention. The fact that there are more people who are witness to disclosure complicates the confidentiality agreement. For instance, members may discuss with each other later what happened in a group supervision session when another colleague is present. The potential for breaches of confidentiality is increased simply because more people are involved.

Working alliance

Bond and Holland (1998, p. 77) note that 'nothing has more influence on the effectiveness of clinical supervision than the quality of the clinical supervision relationship'. The core conditions discussed in Chapter 7 are the foundation for the working alliance. These will take time to develop but it is important to focus on the expectations, preferences, rights and responsibilities of the supervisor and the supervisee at this early stage. A structured and regular review of the relationship can be set up to monitor the working alliance and to raise any difficulties or conflicts. In a group setting these qualities and core conditions need to be openly discussed and agreed as ground rules for the group interactions.

Session format

New supervisees are often unsure of what issues to bring to a supervision session. Time spent early on discussing the types of incidents or aspects of work that are appropriate for clinical supervision will help with this. The basic principle is that supervisees have the responsibility to decide and prepare topics for clinical supervision (Activity 9.3). Bond and Holland (1998) identify four categories of topics that may be selected in preparation, namely, the care of a patient or group of patients; the pressures or stressors emerging from, or influencing, one's work; the areas of responsibility contained in one's work or role; the professional or personal developmental aspects of one's work. Each of these could be explored through reflection on specific incidents or in a more generalised way. The approach, model and style of supervision should also be agreed.

Activity 9.3

Think back over your most recent nursing experience. Select one issue from each of the four categories identified by Bond and Holland (1998) that would be appropriate for your own clinical supervision session:

The care of a specific patient or group of patients.

Pressure(s) or stressors emerging from, or influencing, your work.

An area of responsibility contained in your role.

A professional or personal developmental aspect of your work.

The group supervision contracting requires that a structure is agreed to guide the sessions, ensuring parity of opportunity. For instance, will each member have the chance to present work at each meeting or will there be some form of rota where one or two present their issues at each meeting.

The organisational and professional context

The Trust, unit, agency or department has a vested interest in the clinical supervision process. An organisation may have written a protocol or policy relating to the implementation of clinical supervision and both parties will need to pay attention to this. As previously mentioned, nurses will also have a professional code of conduct. If group supervision takes place with members of other professions, each with their own code of conduct, then this will need to be discussed.

A sixth component that could be added to Hawkins and Shohet's list is evaluation and review. Agreement should be reached as to how the process will be evaluated. An explicit review mechanism will encourage openness in relation to the relationship and the process, prompting modifications to be made where indicated.

FRAMEWORKS FOR CLINICAL SUPERVISION

Cottrell and Smith (2001) observe a proliferation of frameworks, models and approaches to clinical supervision and speculate that this is down to the variety and complexity of nursing. The selection or adaptation of an existing model will be determined by the context, experience and preference of the supervisor in discussion with the supervisee. As Wright et al (1997) suggest it is up to nurses to choose the best model for their specific needs and practice context.

WHAT TO LOOK FOR IN MODELS

Fowler (1996) notes that no one existing model is appropriate for all levels of staff and all clinical specialities. He identifies four desirable elements of a clinical supervision model, namely explicit purpose and function, a focus on the nature of the supervisory relationship, a description of the process and attention to the pragmatics. In addition, a useful model requires flexibility to allow for different contexts and styles and simplicity without excessive reductionism. Each model has its own focus, strengths and limitations. The various clinical supervision models that have been described within the context of nursing may be divided into the following categories.

Developmental models

These are models that attempt to describe and respond to the continuing development of supervisees. They have a dynamic quality in the sense that they encourage the supervision to evolve in line with the experience of the supervisee. Hawkins and Shohet (2000) note that this is the main type of model that has emerged in the USA. These models serve as useful reminders to supervisors to match supervision activity to the skills, knowledge and experience of the supervisee. Examples of these models are Stoltenberg and Delworth (1987), Hawkins and Shohet (2000) and Bond and Holland (1998). They share the structure of stages related to levels of experience. Inexperienced nurses will be more dependent on their supervisors' expertise and be primarily concerned with their roles and how to fulfil them. The task for the supervisor is to provide affirmation and guidance without taking over too much.

In contrast a highly experienced nurse requires a more sophisticated level of reflective dialogue based on consultative support. The heightened level of autonomy is sometimes characterised by what Casement (1985) termed the 'internal supervisor' which refers to an internal processing of clinical events as they happen, similar to Schon's (1983) idea of reflection-in-action. Consequently the supervisee arrives for supervision having already privately processed events and their meaning. The supervisor is required to respond in a distinctively different way and to accept the supervisee as a peer (see examples in Box 9.4). The various theories describe interim steps between the two examples given. One of the challenges for group supervisors is to respond to members who may be at different levels of experience and ensure that all parties remain engaged in the process, either directly or vicariously.

The main strength of developmental models is that they prompt the supervisor to accurately assess the needs of individual supervisees and to plan the supervision to match. They are less helpful in guiding the process and the pragmatics.

Reflective cycle models

A number of models have been described in the nursing literature that provide step-by-step structures for reflection (Gibbs 1988, Johns 1993). Johns' model for reflection on practice is an

---

Box 9.4 Developmental levels of clinical supervision

Supervisee A (newly qualified): 'On my last shift we were really busy and the Sister shouted at me because I made a mistake. I felt so useless but I had never done the procedure on my own before. It's made me think I'm not cut out for this type of nursing.'

Supervisor: 'I can see that this has knocked your confidence. Would it be helpful if we ran over the steps of the procedure together?'

Supervisee B (experienced nurse): 'Things have been fraught on the ward lately and we are all stressed out. The other day Sister criticised the way I did something. At the time I let it go, even though I thought it was unfounded, because of the pressures. I've since thought about it and concluded that the incident reflects a growing conflict between us.'

Supervisor: 'Have you any ideas what this conflict is about?'

example of such a structure that can be used in preparation for, or during, clinical supervision. It consists of six steps (see Box 9.5) which guide the discussion, ending up with a review of learning and consideration of future actions and choices. These models are applicable to specific incidents rather than more general day-to-day issues facing the supervisee. They are attractive to those who prefer a highly structured approach but others may find them over restricting.

Relationship models

Faugier (1992) provides guidelines that focus on the nature and functions of the supervisory relationship. The Growth and Support model defines thirteen characteristics of the relationship, the first letters of which spell out the two words 'GROWTH' and 'SUPPORT' (see Box 9.6).

Faugier (1992) claims that this framework ensures that the supervisor gives sufficient emphasis to all the essential elements of the relationship. It is probably less helpful in guiding the actual process and pragmatics of clinical supervision.

Process models

As the name suggests, these models are frameworks that enable an analysis of the process of clinical supervision. They are useful in understanding the choices that supervisors make and how these impact on the focus of what is discussed. Hawkins and Shohet (2000) describe a 'seven eyed model of supervision' that was originally designed for psychotherapy supervision. It is increasingly used in nursing supervision, particularly in mental health settings. The model uses a double matrix to point out that the task of the supervisory session is to pay attention to the nursing situation. One interesting observation is that the 'client and the work context are carried into the (supervision) session in both the conscious awareness and the unconscious sensing of the supervisee' (Hawkins & Shohet 2000, p. 69). An example of this is known as the parallel process and is illustrated in Box 9.7. The matrices are further subdivided into categories that relate to possible subjects for the supervisor's attention. This concept allows for a more sophisticated reflection of the nurse–patient encounter.

One of the strengths of this model is its flexibility. The depth of reflective analysis can be matched to the developmental stage of the supervisee by focusing on different categories. A possible limitation is the fact that it was designed for psychotherapy and may not fit all nursing contexts.

Integrative models

Some models have been conceived in an attempt to include all aspects of the aforementioned categories. Dexter and Russell (1995) term one such model a client-centred model of supervision. This

---

Box 9.5 A reflective model (Johns 1993)

1. Phenomenon: description of the experience.
2. Causal: the essential contributing factors.
3. Context: significant background features.
4. Reflection: aims, rationale for actions, consequences of actions, feelings, factors influencing actions.
5. Alternative actions: other choices and their consequences.
6. Learning: feelings now, how it could have been improved, learning.

Box 9.6 Growth and support model (Faugier 1992)

Generosity	**S**ensitivity
Rewarding	**U**ncompromising
Openness	**P**ersonal
Willingness to learn	**P**ractical
Thoughtful and thought provoking	**O**rientation
Humanity	**R**elationship
	Trust

Box 9.7 Example of the parallel process in clinical supervision

Supervisee (health visitor): I have been visiting this family for a long time and don't seem to be making any progress with their difficulties. The mother is a single parent and is at the end of her tether with all her problems. Whatever goals we set or advice I give, the mother rejects for one reason or another. I have tried everything and don't know what to do next. I feel so deskilled.

Supervisor: I can't think of any suggestions that you have not already tried. As you were talking I felt myself frantically trying to come up with a solution but have drawn a blank. Like you I am feeling deskilled. I wonder if there is a parallel process going on here. Your client feels helpless and has no idea what to do about her difficult circumstances; you, in turn, now feel helpless because all your attempts to help have come to nothing; you bring your dilemma to me and I experience very similar feelings of helplessness at not coming up with a solution. It is as if the helplessness has been passed along the line.

model outlines the relationship qualities necessary, focuses on the pragmatics and the process, gives attention to the developmental stage of the supervisee, incorporates a reflective problem-solving component and indicates how the model can be applied to different types of supervision. The clear strength of such a model is that it gives attention to all the facets of clinical supervision. The possible limitation is that, in doing so, it becomes overelaborate or restricting through attention to details.

The five categories of models outlined indicate the range of frameworks that are available to nurses. The number of models available is increasing all the time as nurses experiment and adapt the frameworks to fit their own particular contexts and preferences. The responsibility is on supervisors and supervisees to find a model that will inform and guide practice without stifling creativity and versatility.

Supervision groups will also benefit from the adoption of one of these frameworks but the complexity of group behaviour requires additional conceptual understanding. Skilled group facilitators will have cognitive maps that shed light on group development, group process, individual behaviour in groups, potential group conflicts and the group as a help or hindrance to supervision (Inskipp & Proctor 2001).

CLINICAL SUPERVISION AND INTERPERSONAL SKILLS

The premise of this text is that skilled communication is fundamental to effective nursing practice. This equally applies to clinical supervision. The demands made on the clinical supervisor require a range of communication and interpersonal skills, just as the supervisee's ability to articulate their experiences enhances the quality of the exchange. The interpersonal skills used in clinical supervision are transferable skills. In many ways they are the same skills used in the counselling relationships (see Chapter 7). As previously stated, it is the focus of discussion that is different, i.e. clinical supervision is confined to work-related issues, whereas counselling does not have this restriction. Also, the balance and frequency of skills used, for example, suggesting, teaching, information giving are likely to be used in clinical supervision but rarely in counselling.

Reflective skills

Schön (1983) referred to processing experiences as they happen as 'reflection in action' and retrospective reflection after the event as 'reflection on action'. Clinical supervision is a form of structured reflection-on-action in that it takes place after the event, involving a historical processing of experiences. It complements the immediacy of reflection-in-action that experienced nurses use to process events as they happen.

Reflection involves cognitive and emotional components that are expressed through analysis, understanding and catharsis (see pages 76–77). These activities require a degree of introspection that has been observed to be difficult for nurses who exist in a busy world of paying attention to others (Bond & Holland 1998, Dartington 1994). To maximise the potential benefits of clinical supervision nurses have to learn to feel comfortable with this introspective activity both during, and in preparation for, supervision sessions. A model or framework for reflection helps with this.

Feedback skills

Effective feedback promotes self-awareness, increases options, reinforces productive behaviour and encourages the supervisee. The principles of giving and receiving feedback are discussed in Chapter 5 (pages 73–86). These principles are foundational to quality clinical supervision. It is through a balanced and focused dialogue on the supervisee's experiences, decisions, actions and reactions that constructive learning takes place. This balance is achieved through a critical and honest examination of the supervisee's strengths and the identification of areas for further development or alternative choices in practice.

Six category intervention analysis and clinical supervision

Six category intervention analysis (Heron 1990) is discussed briefly in Chapter 5. This framework provides a structure for the analysis of skills used in clinical supervision. The effective supervisor is required to use valid facilitative and authoritative interventions depending on the situation (see Table 9.1). Generally, the more experienced the supervisee the greater the balance will be in favour of facilitative skills. An inexperienced practitioner and supervisee may rely considerably on the advice and suggestions (authoritative) offered by the supervisor, whereas a supervisee with more experience will engage in a more consultative

dialogue that is characterised by the facilitative skills of the supervisor.

Facilitative categories

The majority of the supervisor's interventions are facilitative. These include cathartic, catalytic and supportive categories. They are nondirective ways of helping supervisees to take responsibility for their own learning, decisions and actions. It has been argued that these categories are often appropriate in clinical supervision as they promote ownership and deepen learning (Bond & Holland 1998). The supportive category underpins the supervisory relationship and consists of the core conditions that characterise all of the supervisor's interventions.

Cathartic interventions encourage the expression of emotions that arise from the supervisee's work. The opportunity for the supervisee to translate inner sensations into external expression is thought to be restorative and preferable to the alternative of bottling up one's feelings. Nurses often work with people in stress and distress and the lack of recognition of their own emotional consequences is well documented (McCarthy 1985). In extreme cases the accumulative effects may result in burnout (Maslach 1982). Skilled supervisors notice the emotional consequences of supervisees' work and respond sensitively by encouraging opportunities for catharsis.

Catalytic interventions are foundational in clinical supervision. They serve to draw out information from supervisees in an attempt to clarify understanding, promote self-discovery and reflect on the implications of their experiences. Strategic use of paraphrasing, clarifying, summarising and questioning skills encourage supervisees to reflect aloud on the significance of their nursing experiences.

Authoritative categories

These interventions come from the supervisor's frame of reference. In this sense they are more directive. Prescriptive interventions seek to influence or direct the supervisor's thinking or behaviour.

Table 9.1 Six category intervention analysis (Heron 1990) applied to clinical supervision

Category	Supervisor's actions	Examples
Facilitative		
Cathartic	Helps supervisee to express/release emotions Joys and sorrows of work Debriefing	*'The way he treated you seems so unfair; what would you really like to say to him?'*
Catalytic	Draws out information Encourages self discovery	*'What precisely happened then?'*
Supportive	Affirms the worth of supervisee Encourages and restores Confidence building	*'Over these last few weeks you have had to face some demanding situations but you have coped with them really well'*
Authoritative		
Prescriptive	Makes suggestions Recommends action Directs	*'Perhaps you would like to tell your colleagues about this'*
Informative	Shares knowledge and meaning Gives information	*'I read some research the other day suggesting that ...'*
Confronting	Challenges blind spots, inappropriate attitudes, beliefs actions or commitment Seeks justification Encourages alternative perspectives	*'Have you ever stopped to think why you do it that way?'*

Dexter and Russell (1995) caution against using this type of intervention too early in the reflective cycle. In their view, where it is indicated, it should follow the thinking aloud component described above. Excessive advice, suggestions and directing of behaviour may result in an over-dependence on the supervisor. Having said this, prescriptive interventions clearly have their place, for example, in the case of unsafe practice or with a very inexperienced supervisee. It can be a great relief to new supervisors to realise that they do not always have to come up with neat solutions to each situation that the supervisee brings. It is rare that there is one correct way of responding to any given nursing situation and it is more likely that different alternatives will be explored.

Informative interventions are distinct from prescription in their intention. Information is given in a more neutral style than advice in the sense that it is generally less socially influencing. The crucial factor is judging when information is

appropriate and to resist the temptation for it to become the predominant category. Once again it is likely to be used more often with inexperienced supervisees.

The confronting category is one that most nurses find consistently difficult (Burnard & Morrison 1988, 1991). This seems to be based on a reluctance to challenge others for fear of upsetting them. To be effective clinical supervision needs a tough edge but when delivered constructively a challenge does not alienate or upset the supervisee but prompts a fresh or different perspective. It is certainly true that the term 'confronting' can be interpreted as combative or aggressive in certain situations but within a supervision context this should not be the case. Constructive challenges highlight alternatives and leave the supervisee with something on which to build or to change (Betts 2002). A simple example is asking a supervisee to explain the rationale for a particular nursing action or decision. This often prompts a questioning of nursing practice and results in a deeper reflection on practice.

ADDITIONAL SKILLS REQUIRED OF GROUP SUPERVISORS

The group supervisor requires all of the skills so far identified for one-to-one supervision. In addition the supervision group presents more complex challenges for the supervisor that require extra knowledge and abilities. The group supervisor has to develop the capacity to make sense of the group process, in particular, the mutual influence among group members (see Chapter 6). Any group has a task and a process. In the case of a supervision group the task is to reflect on the members' work-related

Box 9.8 The requirements of group members and the supervisor (Proctor & Inskipp 2001, p. 113)

Requirements of group members:

- to feel safe enough with each other and with the supervisor to trust the group with honest disclosure of their work;
- to have clarity about the task and how this will be worked on;
- to know each other well enough as individuals;
- to accept and respect difference;
- to share values, beliefs and assumptions about human beings, professional helping and groups;
- to have 'good group manners'.

Requirements of the group supervisor:

- to feel comfortable to exercise authority when necessary;
- to have some 'maps' which help the supervisor to understand and act on group process;
- to arrange opportunities for feedback on how the group members are working together.

issues to improve standards, increase learning and support each other. As the group goes about these central functions an emotional life emerges that is unique to this particular combination of individuals. This emotional life or group process will influence everything that happens in the group setting. It will add to the richness of the experience and it will throw up conflicts that may need to be managed by the supervisor. This management will require the application of theoretical maps of group process and the continuous monitoring of group behaviour and interactions.

Responsibility for the success of the group does not rest exclusively with the group supervisor. Proctor and Inskipp (2001) outline the respective requirements of the group members and the group supervisor (Box 9.8). These issues can be discussed early on in the group life when negotiating the modus operandi and ground rules for the group and the group process can be explicitly reviewed on a regular basis as part of the evaluation process.

CONCLUSION

In some countries clinical supervision is slowly becoming established within nursing culture. Ambiguity of the meaning of the term continues to be a problem and may be militating against a wider adoption of clinical supervision in some instances. In particular, the potential for clinical supervision to be confused with other managerial functions is apparent. The diversity of nursing practice means that the principles of clinical supervision will be translated into a variety of types, approaches, styles and formats.

Just like nursing, clinical supervision is an interpersonal process that requires developed communication skills, whether it takes place in a group or a one-to-one setting. Many of these skills are transferable from nursing contexts and include listening and attending, reflection and relationship building. Others may need further training and experience to enable increasing numbers of nurses to function as clinical supervisors.

REFERENCES

Barber P, Norman I 1987 Skills in supervision. Nursing Times 14: 56–57

Betts A 2002 The nurse as communicator. In: Kenworthy N, Snowley G, Gillling C (eds) Common foundation studies in nursing, 3rd ed. Churchill Livingstone, Edinburgh

Betts A, Hanson B 1998 Clinical supervision: Nurses' perceptions of the factors that impact on implementation following a course of preparation for supervisors. University of Nottingham, unpublished evaluation

Blackford J, Street A 1998 The potential of peer clinical supervision to improve nursing practice. Clinical Effectiveness in Nursing 2(4): 205–212

Bond M, Holland S 1998 Skills of clinical supervision for nurses. Open University Press, Buckingham

Burnard P, Morrison P 1988 Nurses' perceptions of their interpersonal skills: A descriptive study using six category intervention analysis. Nurse Education Today 8(5): 266–272

Burnard P, Morrison P 1991 Nurses' interpersonal skills: A study of nurses' perceptions. Nurse Education Today 11(1): 24–29

Butterworth T, Faugier J (eds) 1992 Clinical supervision and mentorship in nursing. Chapman & Hall, London

Butterworth T, Woods D 1998 Clinical governance and clinical supervision; working together to ensure safe and accountable practice. A briefing paper. School of Nursing & Midwifery, University of Manchester, Manchester

Casement P 1985 On learning from the patient. Routledge, London

Cottrell S, Smith G 2001 The development of nursing supervision in the UK. http://www.clinical-supervision.com accessed 12.12.2001

Cutcliffe J, Epling M, Cassedy P, McGregor J, Plant N, Butterworth T 1998 Ethical dilemmas in clinical supervision 2: need for guidelines. British Journal of Nursing 7(16): 978–982

Dartington A 1994 Where angels fear to tread: idealism, despondency and inhibition of thought in hospital nursing. In: Obholzer A, Roberts VZ (eds) The unconscious at work. Routledge, London

Department of Health 1993 A vision for the future: The nursing midwifery and health visiting contribution to health care. HMSO, London

Dexter G, Russell J 1995 Supervision. In: Dexter G, Wash M (eds) Psychiatric nursing skills: A patient centred approach, 2nd edn, pp. 85–95. Chapman & Hall, London

Dexter G, Wash M 1995 Psychiatric nursing skills: A patient centred approach, 2nd edn. Chapman & Hall, London

Faugier J 1992 The supervisory relationship. In: Butterworth T, Faugier J (eds) Clinical supervision and mentorship in nursing. Chapman & Hall, London

Faugier J 1994 Thin on the ground. Nursing Times 90: 64–65

Faugier J 1995 The supervisory relationship. In: Butterworth T, Faugier J (eds) Clinical supervision and mentorship in nursing, pp. 18–36. Chapman & Hall, London

Fish D, Twinn S 1997 Quality clinical supervision. Butterworth-Heinemann, Oxford

Fowler J 1996 How to use models of clinical supervision in practice. Nursing Standard 10(29): 42–47

Gibbs G 1988 Learning by doing: A guide to teaching and learning methods. Further Education Unit. Oxford Polytechnic, Oxford

Hanson B, Betts A 1998 Clinical supervision: Nurses' perceptions of the factors that impact on implementation, following a course of preparation for clinical supervisors. Conference presentation. University of Nottingham School of Nursing Annual Conference, Stoke, Rochford

Hawkins P, Shohet R 2000 Supervision in the helping professions, 2nd edn. Open University Press, Buckingham

Heron J 1990 Helping the client. Sage, London

Inskipp F, Proctor B 2001 Group supervision. In: Scaife J (ed) Supervision in the mental health professions: A practitioner's guide, pp. 99–121. Brunner-Routledge, Hove

Johns C 1993 Professional supervision. Journal of Nursing Management 1: 9–18

King's Fund 1996 The moral maze of practice: A stimulus for reflection and discussion. King's Fund, London

Kohner N 1994 Clinical supervision in practice. King's Fund, London

Maslach C 1982 Burnout: The cost of caring. Prentice Hall, New Jersey

McCarthy P 1985 Burnout in psychiatric nursing. Journal of Advanced Nursing 10: 305–310

Page S, Wosket V 1994 Supervising the counsellor: A cyclical model. Routledge, London

Platt-Koch LM 1986 Clinical supervision for psychiatric nurses. Journal of Psychosocial Nursing 26(1): 7–15

Proctor B 1987 Supervision: A co-operative exercise in accountability. In: Marken M, Payne M (eds)

Enabling and ensuring. National Youth Bureau for Education in Youth and Community Work, Leicester

Proctor B, Inskipp F 2001 Group supervision. In: Scaife J (ed) Supervision in the mental health professions: A practitioner's guide, pp. 99–121. Brunner-Routledge, Hove

Schön DA 1983 The reflective practitioner: how professionals think in action. Temple Smith, London

Smith JP 1995 Clinical supervision: conference by the NHSE. Journal of Advanced Nursing 21(5): 1029–1031

Stoltenberg CD, Delworth U 1987 Supervising counsellors and therapists. Jossey Bass, San Francisco

Swain G 1995 Clinical supervision: The principles and process. Health Visitors Association, London

United Kingdom Central Council for Nursing, Midwifery and Health Visiting 1996 Position statement on clinical supervision for nursing & health visiting. UKCC, London

Wright S, Elliott M, Scholefield H 1997 A networking approach to clinical supervision. Nursing Standard 11(18): 13–41

White E, Butterworth T, Bishop V, Carson J, Jeacock J, Clements A 1998 Clinical supervision: Insider reports of a private world. Journal of Advanced Nursing 28(1): 185–192

FURTHER READING

Bond M, Holland S 1998 Skills of clinical supervision for nurses. Open University Press, Buckingham

Hawkins P, Shohet R 2000 Supervision in the helping professions, 2nd edn. Open University Press, Buckingham

Scaife J 2001 Supervision in the mental health professions: A practitioner's guide. Brunner-Routledge, Hove

http://www.clinical-supervision.com

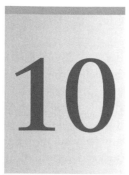

10

Communication and leadership

John Turnbull

INTRODUCTION

This chapter on communication and leadership comes at a significant time both in the development of health services and the careers of nurses. In recent years, the pace of change in the National Health Service (NHS) has increased rapidly, driven mainly by technological developments and a rise in public expectation. Demographic changes, such as an increase in the number of older people in society and people with chronic illness and disabilities, will bring further challenges to those planning and providing health care (Warner et al 1998). At the same time, the aspirations of nurses and expectations of them have been changing and they will continue to do so. There are new opportunities for them to participate in the planning of health care following the creation of Primary Care Trusts (Department of Health 1997), as well as new career opportunities following the introduction of nurse consultants (Department of Health 1999a). Amidst all of this, there will be a continuing need to demonstrate accountability through sound financial management and governance of NHS organisations. If nurses and their colleagues are going to meet these challenges, they will need creative and intelligent leadership.

This chapter aims to improve nurses' understanding of the nature, meaning and purpose of leadership and the role played by communication in helping leaders achieve their aims. The chapter commences by exploring three approaches to understanding leadership. The chapter continues by identifying four main types of leadership and how these different approaches draw upon different forms of communication. The chapter concludes by evaluating the leadership potential of nurses and the opportunities they have to influence others.

THE DIMENSIONS OF LEADERSHIP

 Activity 10.1

Make a list of four people you would consider to be leaders. What do you think makes them stand out as leaders?

For some researchers, leadership is the most important process that takes place in organisations (Rahim 1981). For others, leadership offers the potential to solve countless social problems and ills (Bolman & Deal 1997, p. 294). Practically everyone has experienced leadership in some form. Therefore, it could be stated that leadership is a phenomenon that is a response to universal organisational, social and personal need. Nevertheless, given the breadth of its influence, and the considerable interest shown by researchers, managers, leaders and individuals in the subject, Lancaster (1999) reminded us that there is little agreement on how to define leadership. However, this difficulty provides an opportunity to critically examine the dimensions of leadership in order to identify its key purpose and functions and explore how leaders achieve their goals. Also, although we lack a common definition, we should remember that we have a great deal of knowledge about what leaders do and how they do it.

Since the beginning of systematic enquiry into leadership almost one hundred years ago, there have been three basic approaches to understanding leadership. One of the first beliefs about leaders was that they possessed superior personality traits and characteristics that made them stand out from other people. However, major reviews of research studies into this approach concluded that it was still impossible to identify a set of personality traits that were consistent with effective leadership (Byrd 1940, Jennings 1961). Nevertheless, the feeling that leaders were somehow special prompted other researchers to persist in their efforts to isolate leadership characteristics. Northouse (1997), for example, claimed to have identified five important personality traits that are intelligence, self-confidence, determination, integrity and sociability (pp. 16–18).

Other researchers have placed greater emphasis on what the leader actually does rather than who the leader is. For example, Hersey and Blanchard (1977) have explored the types of skills and competencies that leaders require in order to motivate others. They noticed that leaders were able to adapt their style of leadership to different circumstances. For example, at times, leaders adopted a directive style whereas, at other times, they seemed more supportive. This approach to understanding leadership has become more popular than the trait theory because it implies that leadership behaviour can be learned and, consequently, means that almost anyone could become a leader. It also opened the possibility that there are several styles of leadership, something that we will explore later in this chapter.

Building on the ideas of Hersey and Blanchard, other researchers have proposed that leaders are products of the circumstances that they find themselves in. In other words, the behaviour of leaders is governed primarily by needs of the group or organisation. For many people, this approach makes sense in that an individual or group may only feel the need for leadership at certain times in their development. If this is the case, then the theory suggests that a leader will be identified and will assume responsibility. John Adair (1988) is one of the main proponents of this approach and his 'action-centred' approach to leadership has formed the basis of much leadership training. Although this approach emphasises the primacy of circumstances and group needs, Adair is keen to point out that leaders still require certain skills and characteristics if they are to effectively meet group needs. For example, they need awareness of the needs of the situation, an understanding of what might be needed and the skill to carry out what is required.

Although we lack common agreement on how to understand leadership, one aspect of leadership that everyone agrees upon is that it is strongly linked to the process of communication. As Mullins (1989) states, leadership is a dynamic and interactive process in which leaders require skills in managing relationships with others. If this is the case, then it means that the principles of good communication already outlined in this book will apply to leadership and this will be emphasised in the discussion of different leadership styles. Importantly, we need to recognise that communication between the leader and others will be modified by the many social factors that were discussed in Chapter 3 such as age, gender and ethnicity. Again, as we examine different types of leadership, we will identify how such factors can influence communication.

As well as using these models of communication to understand the function of leadership, the rest of this chapter will also draw upon the work of Bennis and Nanus (1985). Bennis and Nanus believe that leaders are highly competent communicators who manage their interaction with others through

four essential competencies that are briefly described as follows:

◆ Management of attention: knowledge of what is important and what others should be focusing upon.
◆ Management of meaning: how the leader articulates and communicates what is important.
◆ Management of trust: how the leader develops their relationship with others and how the leader manages others' perceptions of the leader's qualities.
◆ Management of self: how the leader communicates their values to others.

This chapter examines the similarities and differences in how these competencies are applied to four different leadership functions and the matrix in Table 10.1 provides a snapshot of this. The four categories of leadership are taken from an analysis of leadership style and function by Bolman and Deal (1997). Their analysis is similar to other descriptions of leadership styles, but this has been chosen because it is comprehensive, up-to-date and

Table 10.1 Leadership type and communication competency

Leadership type/ communication competency	Structural	Visionary	Empowering	Symbolic
MANAGING ATTENTION	'I know what is important'		'You know what is important'	
MANAGING MEANING	The leader 'tells' people what needs to happen	The leader 'sells' the idea by persuasion and negotiation	The leader creates meaning by giving information and supporting others to shape the idea into action	The leader creates meaning through his or her actions or through symbolic ways
MANAGING TRUST	Leader creates trust by acting as a 'parent'	Leader creates trust through his or her expertise and better knowledge	Leader acts as an experienced 'coach'	Leader acts as a role model for others or catalyst for action
MANAGING SELF	Respect is expected because of position of authority	Respect is given to others		

informed by the authors' personal experience and insight into the running of organisations. Having said this, their descriptions have been adapted for the purposes of this chapter.

Structural leadership

The first type of leadership we will explore is what Handy (1993) and Bolman and Deal (1997) have referred to as structural leadership. Structural leaders invariably occupy positions of authority in their organisations and this is a key factor in understanding how this type of leadership works. For example, Abraham and Shanley (1992) have pointed out that having a senior position in an organisation can play a significant role in establishing someone's credentials as a leader in the eyes of other people. Likewise, a person in a position of authority is more likely to have expectations that he or she will show leadership to others. To understand this in terms of a communication process, it perhaps confirms the importance of perception, in that greater importance will be attributed to the words and actions of people in positions of authority.

Largely because of the legitimacy that their position confers on them, structural leaders possess a powerful belief in the importance of their ideas and plans for organisations. In terms of the leadership competencies shown in Table 10.1, this could be understood as them having an unshakeable belief that they know what is important for the organisation and the people who work in it. This can also be inferred from the way that structural leaders communicate their idea to others. For example, Hersey and Blanchard (1988, p. 177) compared styles of communication to different types of leaders and concluded that structural leaders adopt a 'telling' style. In other words, their communication was high on giving directions and instructions and low on listening. Structural leaders were also reluctant to share information, probably because of their belief that this might result in alternatives to their own solutions. They were also less likely to want to share problems with others because they

believed that this might result in them being perceived as weak or indecisive.

From the description of structural leaders given so far, we might conclude that such individuals are more akin to autocrats and bullies than leaders. However, research provides evidence that this type of leadership can be highly effective in certain circumstances. Furthermore, Bolman and Deal (1997) have provided case examples from several national and multinational companies to show that structural leadership can sometimes be welcomed by organisations. Studies by White and Lippit (1968) have shown that groups whose leaders dictated their policies and allocated tasks were more productive than groups in which leaders adopted a more participative approach. However, the researchers also found that there was more aggression and dependence in the groups who had more directive leaders. A similar set of experiments conducted by Fiedler (1967) has produced evidence that leaders who were more directive tended to focus the group's activities on the task to be done with the result that they were more productive than groups with leaders who were more person-focused. Interestingly, in an experiment with air-force personnel, Fiedler also discovered that leaders who became more 'distant' in their interaction with their subordinate officers succeeded in improving their productivity. Fiedler explains this phenomenon thus:

> 'When he (the officer) had very close relations with these officers, they seemed to feel secure and they did not worry overly about the efficiency of their units. As soon as he became more reserved and role-orientated, his sub-commanders began to worry whether anything had gone awry. They became less secure about their standing in the organisation, and channelled their anxieties into paying more attention to their work. As a result, there was a noticeable increase in the efficiency of the base'. (Cited in Handy 1993, p. 105).

Although there are inconsistencies in the research on productivity and leadership style, Abraham and

Shanley's (1992) review of the literature concluded that, under certain circumstances, a directive, or structural style of leadership may be more appropriate, albeit on a short-term basis. For example, an overspend on the bank and agency staff budget in a hospital might be resolved if a senior manager was the only person allowed to authorise expenditure. Also, in a relatively stable environment, a directive style of leadership can assist in keeping employees 'on task'. In contrast, the authors also point out that, when a group is under pressure and has few resources, a directive leader may be welcomed because he or she will relieve others from the responsibility of decision-making. Likewise, in many crisis situations, groups will look to someone to show them the way quickly. This point is often used to explain why wartime leaders are relatively ineffective in peacetime, or even why some football managers achieve greater success when clubs are threatened by relegation and vice-versa. Handy (1993) added to this by stating that we cannot deny that some people in organisations prefer to be directed and have relatively low needs to be independent. He cited the example of Douglas McGregor who, despite his beliefs in a more democratic style of management, discovered that he had to play the role of the 'boss' (see Box 10.1). Furthermore, he stated that, in organisations in which repetitive and routine work is the norm, a structured approach might be more effective in maintaining productivity. It is arguable whether productivity could be increased in the longer term using a different approach. However, a conclusion must be that different circumstances give rise to the need for different types of leaders.

Activity 10.2

Given what we know about the benefits of a structural approach to leadership, are there any areas of nursing practice or circumstances in nursing in which a structural approach could be beneficial?

Box 10.1 Structural leadership

Douglas McGregor has written many books on the subject of leadership and management. When he left the Antioch College, of which he had been president, he announced, '*I believed that a leader could operate successfully as a kind of adviser to his organisation. I thought I could avoid being a "boss"… I thought that maybe I could operate so that everyone would like me – that good human relations would eliminate all discord and disagreement. I couldn't have been more wrong. It took a couple of years, but I finally began to realise that a leader cannot avoid the exercise of authority any more than he can avoid the responsibility for what happens in his organisation*' (cited in Handy 1993, p. 101)

In terms of health care, the idea of productivity and a task-oriented approach might seem alien. Therefore, it is difficult to imagine how structural leadership could be applied. However, the recent introduction of modern matrons into the NHS could be seen as a recognition of the need for a more authoritative and decisive form of leadership in some areas of health care practice (Department of Health 2001). It could also be seen as a recognition by government that areas of NHS provision are in crisis. For example, modern matrons are charged with providing 'a visible, accessible and authoritative presence in ward settings to whom patients and their families can turn to for assistance, advice and support.' (Department of Health 2001). Guidance also directs NHS Trusts to ensure that modern matrons have sufficient authority to ensure 'that the basics of care' are right and that they have the authority to ensure that wards are cleaned appropriately. The Department of Health acknowledges that modern matrons may be more applicable to in-patient areas than community settings that are more multidisciplinary and multiagency in their practice.

Although it is important that the Department of Health has recognised the need for different approaches to leadership, and that a structural approach to leadership can have benefits, it is equally important that local managers take account of the evidence and experience of this type of leadership. For example, Bolman and Deal (1997) have rightly pointed out that every style of leadership has its disadvantages if applied inappropriately. In the case of structural leaders, individuals can turn into petty tyrants and dictators if they use the authority of their position alone to get things done. Furthermore, as shown above, structural leaders may be more effective in the short-term in sorting out a crisis and it may take another form of leadership to maintain any gains that are made.

Visionary leadership

Activity 10.3

Think of an area of practice that you want to change. Whose support would you need to make the change and how would you persuade them to support you?

A consistent theme in the literature on leadership is that leaders are expected to have a vision of the future and are able to give direction to others (Covey 1992, Kotter 1990). In recent studies, that have asked people what they look for in a leader, this continues to be a powerful theme (Alimo-Metcalfe & Alban-Metcalfe 2000, Jones 2001). Precisely what enables leaders to develop their visions has also been the subject of considerable investigation and the answer seems to lie both in their personal characteristics as well as the circumstances they find themselves in. For example, Gardner (1989) concluded that visionary leaders have a capacity to think long-term and to question their own as well as others' assumptions about the world in which they live and work. This allows them to think outside of traditional boundaries and to develop a view of how different things could be. The context of change is equally important in supporting the

visionary leader. In their exploration of leadership, Hersey and Blanchard (1988) concluded that visionary leadership is more successful when the people who are being influenced possess the motivation to change but lack knowledge about precisely what needs changing or how this could happen.

In terms of managing the attention of others, visionary leadership is similar to structural leadership, in that it is the leader who must have the idea as well as a belief in what is right for others and the organisation. However, the way this is communicated is significantly different. Having a vision of the future does not have to depend on someone's position in an organisation. Therefore, whereas structural leaders can use their position in an organisation to 'tell' people what must happen, visionary leaders must enlist the support of others and 'sell' their ideas. This calls for individuals who can negotiate with and persuade others of their ideas.

Jay Conger, Professor of Organisational Behaviour at the University of Southern Carolina in the United States, has spent a great deal of time observing and interviewing business managers and leaders to understand how they negotiate and persuade others to support their ideas. In one of his articles about his research, Conger (1998) has described how, and how not, to use persuasion. Conger's first piece of advice for would-be persuaders is the need to establish credibility with the people they are trying to influence. On a psychological level, Conger explains that allowing us to be persuaded is a risk because any initiative demands our commitment, time and resources. Therefore, someone is more likely to take this risk for someone who is perceived as possessing expert knowledge and experience. This factor is consistently supported by other research. For example, in a recent study in a NHS Trust, a range of staff was asked to list the factors of a good leader (Jones 2001). Almost all staff reported that 'trustworthiness' and 'expertise' were essential characteristics. Another important factor in Conger's investigation was the quality of the relationship between the leader and those being influenced. Conger points out that a major mistake that people often make when trying to persuade others is to believe that persuasion is a one-off event. Conger points out that persuasion uses a variety of communication skills:

'Even before starting to persuade, the best persuaders ... use conversations, meetings and other forms of dialogue to collect essential information. They are good at listening. They test out their ideas with trusted confidants, and they ask questions of the people they will later be persuading. Those steps help them to think through the arguments, the evidence and the perspectives they will present.'
(Conger 1998)

Again, Conger's ideas are supported by other research that has shown that effective leaders are often people with an extensive network of contacts (Meindl 1990). Keeping in touch with networks enables the individual to be in a better position to persuade when the time arises. Conger also points out that the leader must be prepared to compromise. Again, on a psychological level, a person who shows that they cannot compromise gives the message that they think persuasion is a one-way process in which one party must give in. This does not mean that the leader must abandon their vision: often, other people's ideas can modify an idea and turn it into a more workable solution to a problem (see Box 10.2). Finally, Conger points out that people often make the mistake of believing that persuasion depends upon presenting powerful arguments. He points out that the leader must be sensitive to the context in which they find themselves. Bennis et al (1976) have taken up this point in their discussion of different strategies for change management. They identified three distinct approaches that are summarised in Box 10.3. One of these strategies, the rational–empirical approach, is based on the assumption that people are basically rational people who will be prepared to change if presented with a logical argument. Conger believes that presenting evidence is important in any argument. However, he notes that it may be insufficient in helping people to change and needs to be supported by language

---

Box 10.2 Visionary leadership in nursing

'I had been telling the RCN for some time about the differences between learning disability nursing and psychiatry. Until 1983 both groups were represented on a joint RCN committee with four learning disability members and twenty from mental health. While relationships were good between the two groups, those from learning disability were outnumbered in everything. The breakthrough came when Trevor Clay went to the RCN Council and got some money for the learning disability adviser's post. He said to me "Well, you've been moaning about the situation for some time – put your money where your mouth is and apply for the post". I did, and I got the job. It was the best thing that I ever did.' (McMillan 1999).

'A nurse on a psychiatric ward provided leadership after listening to a group of patients on her ward talk about the lack of dignity shown to them by the hospital. Working with the patients, the nurse arranged for a special meal to be organised in recognition of the patients' desire to be valued. The meal involved a nicely set table and well presented food which was to be served by the qualified staff and health care assistants. The nurse had to work hard at persuading managers to release the money involved in providing extra resources. The most challenging aspect was winning the support of the health care assistants who initially resented the idea of any of the staff 'serving' the food to the patients. The nurse listened to the concerns of the health care assistants, acknowledging their difficulty in making this small yet significant change to their practice. Eventually, it was agreed that a 'trial' meal would take place. The patients were very pleased to receive the meal and responded more positively to the ward staff. The health care assistants appreciated the more congenial attitude from the patients towards them. The nurse is now working towards looking at how patients and the staff can work together in making the ward environment a better place to be.' (Ewens 2002).

Box 10.3 Strategies for change (from Bennis et al 1976)

Power–coercive: The change agent relies on the authority of their position and makes the assumption that others will follow those in authority. The change agent provides information, gives orders, directs change and defines the who, what, where, when and how of the change process.

Rational–empirical: This approach is based on the assumption that people are rational and that they will make judgements on the merits of argument. The change agent provides information and attempts to convince others of the need for change. The change agent provides support for change but is less directive than the power–coercive approach.

Normative–re-educative: This approach assumes that people will want to be involved in the process of change. The change agent negotiates with others in decision-making. Information and directions can be provided when asked for by others.

and images that connect with people on an emotional level:

> 'Ordinary evidence won't do. We have found that the most effective persuaders use language in a particular way. They supplement numerical data with examples, stories, metaphors, and analogies to make their positions come alive.' (Conger 1998)

Jay Conger's advice on how to communicate with others and persuade them more closely resembles an educational rather than an adversarial process. It also shows us that, in persuading others to adopt their vision, leaders must give respect to those they are trying to convince. Finally, in order to establish trust and credibility, leaders must be perceived as having particular expertise. Given this analysis, the recent introduction of nurse consultants in the NHS appears to be an initiative aimed at creating visionary leaders within the profession (Department of Health 1999a). In its circular announcing the introduction of nurse consultants, the Department of Health (1999a) set out four essential functions for nurse consultants that are:

◆ an expert practice function;
◆ a professional leadership and consultancy function;
◆ an education, training and development function;
◆ a practice and service development, research and evaluation function.

Activity 10.4

Given the remit of nurse consultants outlined above, what problems do you think they will encounter in fulfilling their leadership role?

Although these posts are in their early days, preliminary evaluation has already highlighted positive features as well as challenges in putting them into practice (Guest et al 2001). As far as current discussion is concerned, nurse consultants report problems in establishing their credibility with others. We have already seen how perceptions play an important role in the communication process and it could be that more traditional images of nurses as being subservient to medical roles are playing a part in the lack of acceptance of nurse consultants. On the other hand, nursing colleagues may be playing their part in the problems that nurse consultants are experiencing by expecting too much from these posts.

As with other types of leadership, visionary leadership can be inappropriately applied. Bolman and Deal (1997) have noted that visionary leaders can sometimes be perceived as idealists. This accusation is more likely to be made when the leader lacks credibility. Visionary leaders also run the risk of being seen as too dogmatic. Again, this may happen if the leader is reluctant to listen to others and to compromise.

Empowering leadership

Imagine that we are observing a conversation between a ward sister and a staff nurse on a ward. The sister has noticed that the staff nurse has not contributed as much as she usually does to the nursing team meetings and that she seems demotivated. During the conversation the staff nurse reveals that she has been thinking of applying for a sister's post on another ward. The staff nurse doesn't want to let down the rest of the team, which partly explains her reticence in recent meetings. However, she is also wondering whether she is ready for the promotion and responsibility.

Activity 10.5

Imagine that you are the sister in this scenario. What might you be feeling and what would you want to communicate to the staff nurse during the rest of the conversation?

Naturally, the sister is disappointed that she might lose an important member of her team. However, she realises that she must act to develop the confidence of her colleague. She asks the staff nurse to recall how she felt when she first got her staff nurse's job on the ward. The sister also asks the staff nurse to recall times when she has deputised for the sister and how she felt. Finally, the ward sister asks the staff nurse to list the qualities that she feels she will bring to a ward sister's post. By the end of the conversation, the staff nurse feels more confident and aware of her motives for becoming a ward sister and she is determined to apply for the vacant post.

In this brief example, we can see a third type of leadership in action. In contrast to visionary leadership, in which one person tries to convince others of the merits of their ideas, the ward sister has helped her colleague to develop her own vision for her future and to summon-up the courage to put it into practice. This type of leadership is often referred to as empowering leadership. Like other types of leadership, this approach is made effective when the circumstances are right as well as when the leader demonstrates the right qualities. Hersey and Blanchard (1988) have noted that this type of leadership is most effective in situations in which an individual, or group, is able and knowledgable but is insecure and, therefore, lacks motivation. In the example above, the staff nurse felt uncertain about putting her ideas into practice. This may apply equally to some patients and clients that we come across. For example, people with learning disabilities can have clear ideas about how they want to live their lives but may lack confidence in making decisions. Other writers have attributed the interest in and need for empowering leadership to social change, in that people now demand greater control over their lives (Brotherton 1999). Turnbull (2002) also believes that changes in the workplace have set the conditions for empowering leadership to flourish. This is because our economy has moved away from manufacturing, in which the tasks of workers need to be directed, towards a service-led economy that demands greater creativity and imagination from employees.

As far as the qualities of the empowering leader are concerned, their main role is to provide the motivation and to instil confidence in others. In contrast to the previous types of leadership, empowering leadership is firmly based on the assumption that other people know what is important and, because of this, the leader's actions must convey trust and respect for others. Nancy Kline (1999), an international leadership consultant, has developed a process for organisations to become more empowering that she calls 'The Thinking Environment' (Thinking Environment is a registered trademark). The ten components of the Thinking Environment are shown in Box 10.4. Kline believes that the cornerstone of respecting others is the quality of

> **Box 10.4** The 10 components of a Thinking Environment (adapted from Kline 1999)
>
> 1. **Attention.** The quality of your attention determines the quality of other people's thinking.
>
> 2. **Equality.** Treat each other as thinking peers. Even in a hierarchy people can be equals as thinkers.
>
> 3. **Ease.** Ease creates and urgency destroys. When it comes to helping people think for themselves, sometimes doing means not doing.
>
> 4. **Encouragement.** Move beyond competition. To be 'better than' is not necessarily to be good.
>
> 5. **Appreciation.** Practice a 5:1 ratio of praise to criticism. The human mind processes criticism best in a context of concrete, genuine praise.
>
> 6. **Feelings.** Allowing sufficient emotional release to restore thinking. Fear constricts everything. Crying can make you smarter.
>
> 7. **Information.** Supply the truth. Withholding information results in intellectual vandalism.
>
> 8. **Incisive questions.** Remove assumptions that limit ideas.
>
> 9. **Place.** Create a physical environment that says back to people, 'you matter'.
>
> 10. **Diversity.** The mind thinks best in the presence of reality. Reality is diverse. Therefore, homogeneity is a form of denial.

attention that we give and that good attention requires good listening. However, Kline believes that listening is a communication skill that is in short supply:

'We think we listen, but we don't. We finish each other's sentences, we interrupt each other, we moan together, we fill in the pauses with our own stories, we look at our watches, sigh, frown, tap our finger, read the newspaper, or walk away. We give advice, give advice and give advice. Even professional listeners listen poorly much of the time. They come in too soon with their own ideas. They equate talking with looking professional.' (Kline 1999, p. 37).

Kline later expanded on her point about some of the risks in employing an 'active listening' style that professionals are traditionally taught to use:

'Real help, professionally or personally, consists of listening to people, of paying respectful attention to people so that they can access their own ideas first. Usually, the brain that contains the problem also contains the solution – often the best one. When you keep that in mind, you become more effective with people. And people around you end up with better ideas. This is not to say that advice is never a good thing or that your ideas are never needed. Sometimes your suggestions are exactly what the person wants and needs ... But don't rush into it. Give people a chance to find their own ideas first' (Kline 1999, p. 39).

As well as listening, Nancy Kline also proposed that people are encouraged to think for themselves better by the skilled use of questions. Kline believes that many people are discouraged from putting forward and developing their ideas because of assumptions they hold. Typically, assumptions that can limit someone's thinking include, 'My ideas aren't as good as other people's', 'My ideas won't make a difference' or 'I don't deserve success'. Kline described how a skilful leader can remove these assumptions by posing questions that replace the limiting assumption with one that frees them to think more creatively as well as to focus them on the key issue or problem. For example, in answer to the assumptions above, possible questions include, 'If you knew that you are as intelligent as your bosses, how would you present yourself to them?' or 'If you knew you were vital to the organisation's success, how would you approach your work?'

In their evaluation of implementing patient-centred nursing into an acute ward, Binnie and Titchen (1999) confirmed the importance of good listening and questioning on behalf of the leader to encourage openness, curiosity and learning amongst a team of nurses. Here, one of the nurses described its impact:

> 'Alison opens our ideas to new ideas, new ways of looking at things ... When she takes an interest in our patients, she says, "Have you thought of this or that?" She makes me think about a much wider area than I have been used to. During handover, she will ask questions about the patient, about things that I hadn't really thought about.' (Binnie & Titchen 1999, p. 112).

Likewise, Ann Ewens (2002) has described how an empowering approach to learning was introduced into a Master's degree level module on leadership. Ewens attributed its success to the quality of listening and attention displayed by students and tutors as well as the use of questions to encourage reflection on practice.

Once again, the empowering approach to leadership can create risks in organisations if it is not applied appropriately and skilfully. For example, Bolman and Deal (1997) noted that empowering leaders can be perceived as paying too little attention to tasks that need to be carried out in an organisation. Others may believe that empowering leaders can be too permissive, and, by encouraging individuality, that their approach could lead to chaos in organisations.

Symbolic leadership

So far, the three types of leadership that we have discussed suggest that a combination of qualities, skills and circumstances interact to ascribe both roles of leaders and followers to people in organisations. Symbolic leadership offers a different perspective on the topic and, because of this, its characteristics and assumptions do not fit neatly into the categories originally outlined in Table 10.1. Christopher Spence, the founder of the London Lighthouse for people with HIV/AIDS, is someone who invites us to look in other directions for leadership:

> 'We must assume the leadership of everyone. Leadership is to do with being human, rather than with having people to lead ... If you think about it, our nature is to lead. We lead our lives, making sure things go well for us and those about us. We share who we are and what we have. We beautify the environment. We step forward for what we believe in and value. We speak up, to influence, attract, inspire. We tell the truth. We care. We love. We dream. These natural expressions of our humanity are, in fact, the foundations of real leadership.' (Spence 1996, p. 57).

This is a highly inclusive and radical view of leadership. In terms of our previous discussion in this chapter it suggests that we could look for leadership in a 10-year-old child and a person with learning disabilities as well as a chief executive of an NHS Trust or a ward sister. Of course, if we accept a traditional view of the leader as privileged and someone to follow, then if everyone is a leader, no-one is a leader. As far as organisations are concerned, this seems like a recipe for chaos and anarchy. However, if we view leadership as something that inspires and energises, then it opens up infinite possibilities for organisations and the people who work in them.

Continuing his discussion, Spence has suggested that our current view of leadership is an artificial and limiting construct that arises out of our negative experiences of our upbringing and the organisations we go on to work in. He explained:

> 'As children we wanted things to be right. We wanted harmony, co-operation, progress, respect, justice, truth, well-being. We led until we had to surrender to the incessant blows of ridicule, caution, confusion, the low sights of those influencing us. So, we arrive at

adulthood doubting our leadership, assuming only a chosen few can lead and setting limits on our sphere of influence in the world. We are probably deterred too by the way we see leaders behave, lest we be thought to be presuming, or assuming a role perceived to be hurtful.' (Spence 1996, pp. 57–58).

In the previous types of leadership we have explored, the assumption is that the leader develops characteristics and acquires skills to perform a leadership function. In contrast, Spence's view assumes that leaders must discard ways of thinking and behaving, such as fear and competitiveness, and reconnect with innate qualities such as respect and co-operation. Therefore, this type of leadership is not so much a way of *doing* but a way of *being* in the world. In terms of a communication process, we can be inspired by our direct contact with other people. For example, we might admire the dignity and resilience of the 80-year-old woman patient who has spent much of her life in a long-stay hospital. We can also admire the courage of the 10-year-old boy preparing for his fifth heart operation. Spence's view of leadership also makes it possible for people to communicate and offer leadership in more symbolic forms. For example, we can be moved by music, literature and other art forms. Spence's ideas

also go some way to explain the impact that a high-profile individual can have on us. For example, the late Princess of Wales is someone who many people found inspirational. Although we have to acknowledge that our impressions of her were mediated through the television and newspapers, she is frequently mentioned when people discuss leadership (see Box 10.5).

Whether perceptions such as Nancy Kline's described in Box 10.5 are accurate, society perhaps needs people who seem to represent key values and qualities. The word 'role-model' is over-used and inadequate to describe many of these people. The danger is that such people are given the status of heroes and heroines. This would be to contradict the basic assumption of symbolic leadership that is that everyone holds equal status.

Activity 10.6

Consider Christopher Spence's description of leadership given above and the discussion that followed. What would be the impact on the area of practice that you work in of assuming this view of leadership?

LEADERSHIP AND NURSING

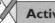

Activity 10.7

Given what you have learned about leadership style, do you think that there is one style of leadership that is more appropriate for nurses to use?

Box 10.5 Symbolic leadership in action. The example of Diana, Princess of Wales

'On many occasions I watched her give unfailingly the highest calibre attention to people. I watched her look into their eyes, bend one knee slightly, rest her arms easily in front of her, relax and listen as if they were the only person in the world at that moment. Often she had literally only a moment, but in a split second, because of the quality of her attention, she disarmed feelings of nervousness and assumptions of inferiority and allowed people to remember that they matter'. (Kline 1999, p. 250)

Most writers agree that the type of leadership that nurses have experienced has been a controlling and directive one that has had a negative impact on nursing practice (Ewens 2002, Traynor 1999). For example, Keen and Malby (1992) have investigated the impact of the introduction of general management in the health service on nurses and concluded that many had lost power to nonprofessional managers. Stewart (1996) has also noted how nursing has consistently been viewed as being subordinate to the medical profession. Furthermore, with its emphasis on control and competition, Cook (1999) and Lancaster (1999) concluded that the style of leadership and management within the NHS over the past 30 years is a highly 'masculine' approach. Therefore, the fact that nursing is a predominantly female profession has put nurses at a disadvantage in assuming power and influence in organisations. Wells (1999) has expanded on this point by observing that nurses have merely copied a hierarchical and controlling style of management at ward level.

As we have seen from the discussion of leadership styles, the directive approach to management can be useful, if applied appropriately, to relatively stable conditions. However, the current context in which health practitioners find themselves is more turbulent. Commissioning and providing health care is also likely to become more complex. Ferlie and Pettigrew (1996) have pointed to the need to see health care provision as a system requiring the collaboration of partner organisations and different agencies. This will require a different type of leadership that encourages networking, partnership working and leaders who can think beyond their immediate organisational and professional boundaries and can manage relationships intelligently and skilfully. It will also require all of the people who work in health services to be able to respond quickly to change and who can plan and execute improvements in their sphere of practice.

A key question is how well equipped are nurses to play a full role in leading change in a modernised NHS? On a strategic level, the Department of Health has recognised the need to strengthen nursing leadership in a new strategy for nursing (Department of Health 1999b). Two significant changes that have occurred as a result of this document are the introduction of modern matrons and nurse

consultant posts. As we have already discussed, modern matrons will be responsible for ensuring that the basics of care are provided in ward areas and that they will have sufficient authority to ensure a clean and safe environment for patients and staff. Nurse consultants are expected to be more visionary and creative, and to provide clinical leadership within and outside their profession. These innovations should be welcomed, especially if they help to change the way that others perceive nurses and nursing leaders. However, nursing leadership should not be the preserve of a handful of nurses with particular titles. Wedderburn-Tate (1999) observed that nurses demonstrate many leadership skills and qualities in their daily practice that go unnoticed. The humanistic foundations of nursing practice, such as unconditional respect and valuing of others is not only at the heart of person-centred nursing practice but is central to empowering and symbolic leadership styles. For example, nurses frequently find themselves collaborating with patients and clients in order to help them arrive at solutions to physical and emotional difficulties that are right for them. The communication skills that nurses need to use in their daily interactions with patients and clients such as listening and giving information and explanations clearly are also skills needed by leaders in persuading and negotiating with others. Finally, as the health service works to become a more person-centred organisation that builds its services around the needs and wishes of the public, it should not be forgotten that nurses possess considerable information about those needs. Therefore, nurses are in a position to play a full role in developing a vision for the future.

CONCLUSION

This chapter has shown that leadership is a complex phenomenon that comprises a number of different styles in which the leader is expected to demonstrate a range of qualities and skills. The context in which leadership is offered is also significant in determining which style of leadership is appropriate. Above all, leadership is an interactive process that draws upon the full range of communication skills. It has been argued that nurses already demonstrate a range of leadership skills which will become more important to the health service and those who use it as the NHS modernises its structure and practice.

REFERENCES

Abraham C, Shanley E 1992 Social psychology for nurses. Edward Arnold, London

Adair J 1988 The Action Centred Leader. Industrial Society, London

Alimo-Metcalfe B, Alban-Metcalfe R 2000 Heaven can wait. Health Service Journal 12th October: 26–29

Bennis WG, Benne KD, Chin R, Corey KE 1976 The planning of change. Holt, Reinhart and Winston, London

Bennis WG, Nanus B 1985 Leaders: the strategies for taking charge. Harper Row, New York

Binnie A, Titchen A 1999 Freedom to practise: the development of patient centred nursing. Butterworth Heinemann, Oxford

Bolman LG, Deal TE 1997 Reframing organisations: artistry, choice and leadership, 2nd edn. Jossey Bass, San Francisco

Byrd C 1940 Social psychology. Appleton-Century-Crofts, New York

Conger J 1998 The necessary art of persuasion. Harvard Business Review May–June: 84–95

Cook M 1999 Improving care requires leadership in nursing. Nurse Education Today 19: 306–312

Covey SR 1992 The seven habits of highly effective people. Simon and Schuster, London

Department of Health 1997 The new NHS: modern, dependable. Department of Health, London

Department of Health 1998 A first class service. Department of Health, London

Department of Health 1999a Nurse consultant posts. HSC1999/217. Department of Health, London

Department of Health 1999b Making a difference. Strengthening the nursing, midwifery and health visiting contribution to health and healthcare. Department of Health, London

Department of Health 2000 The NHS plan. Department of Health, London

Department of Health 2001 Implementing the NHS plan: modern matrons. Strengthening the role of ward sisters and introducing senior sisters. HSC 2001/10. Department of Health, London

Department of Health and Social Security 1983 National Health Service management enquiry. HMSO, London

Ewens A 2002 The nature and purpose of leadership. In: Howkins E, Thornton C (eds) Managing and leading innovation in healthcare. Ballière Tindall, London

Ferlie E, Pettigrew A 1996 Managing through networks: some issues and implications for the NHS. British Journal of Management 7: 81–99

Fiedler FEA 1967 A theory of leadership effectiveness. McGraw-Hill, New York

Gardner JW 1989 On leadership. Free Press, New York

Guest D, Redfern S, Wilson-Barnett J et al 2001 A preliminary investigation of the establishment of nurse, midwife and health visitor consultants. University of London, London

Ham C 1992 Health policy in Britain, 3rd edn. MacMillan, Basingstoke

Handy C 1993 Understanding organisations, 4th edn. Penguin, Harmondsworth

Hersey P, Blanchard K 1977 Management of organisational behaviour, 3rd edn. Prentice-Hall, Englewood Cliffs, New Jersey

Hersey P, Blanchard K 1988 Management of organisational behaviour, 5th edn. Prentice-Hall, Englewood Cliffs, New Jersey

Jennings EE 1961 The anatomy of leadership. Management of Personnel Quarterly 1(1): 2

Jones H 2001 Towards leadership development. Unpublished M.Sc thesis in Human Resource Management, Oxford

Keen J, Malby R 1992 Nursing power and practice in the United Kingdom National Health Service. Journal of Advanced Nursing 17: 863–870

Kline N 1999 Time to think: listening to ignite the human mind. Ward Lock, London

Kotter J 1990 A force for change. Collier MacMillan, London

Lancaster J 1999 Nursing issues in managing and leading change. Mosby Inc., Missouri

McMillan I 1999 Still knocking 'em for six after all these years. Profile of Alan Parrish. Learning Disability Practice 1(4): 4–5

Mullins L 1989 Management and organisational behaviour, 2nd edn. Pitman, London

Northouse P 1997 Leadership: theory and practice. Sage, London

Rahim A 1981 Organisational behaviour course for graduate students in business administration: views from the tower and the battlefield. Psychological Reports 49: 583–592

Spence C 1996 On watch: views from the lighthouse. Cassell, London

Stewart R 1996 Leading in the NHS: a practical guide. Macmillan, Basingstoke

Traynor M 1999 Managerialism and nursing: beyond oppression and profession. Routledge, London

Turnbull J 2002 Managing to change the way we manage to change. In: Howkins E, Thornton C (eds) Managing innovation and creativity in healthcare. Ballière Tindall, London

Warner M, Longley M, Gould E, Pieck A 1998 Healthcare futures 2010. UKCC, London

Wells JSG 1999 The growth of managerialism and its impact on nursing and the NHS. In: Norman I, Cowley S (eds) The changing nature of nursing in a managerial age. Blackwell Science, Oxford

White R, Lippit R 1968 Leader behaviour and member reaction in three 'social climates'. In: Cartwright D, Zander A (eds) Group dynamics: theory and research. Tavistock, London

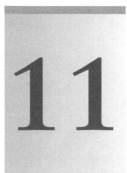

11

Communicating with the wider world

Debra Moore

INTRODUCTION

This chapter examines the role of the nurse when communicating in the wider world of health and social care.

In the context of this chapter the 'wider world' includes teams, agencies, forums, statutory bodies, local and national organisations; all of whom the nurse may find themself working with, and alongside, to improve patient care.

Developments over recent decades have seen health care delivery in much of the Western world move from traditional hospital settings and outpatient clinics, to primary care centres and community-based teams. This movement in the focus of health care looks set to continue due to the political and patient demands to cut hospital waiting lists, shorten the length of stay in hospital and provide rehabilitation at home. Additionally, the 'mixed economy' of care created in the 1980s by Conservative Party policy has meant that, as a practitioner, you may be providing nursing care in a variety of settings, and interfacing with any number of organisations.

Shifts in the location of care delivery have also created a widening effect in relation to the number of people and agencies involved in any one person's care. It can be seen that when the patient is cared for in hospital the different professionals or 'providers' of care are usually employed by one organisation for example an NHS Trust rather than when the person is nursed at home, where the number of people may be greater or fewer, but the organisations they work for may be many. This is illustrated in Figure 11.1.

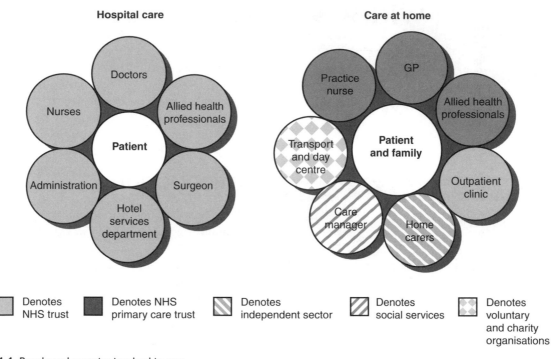

Fig 11.1 People and agencies involved in care

To accommodate such changes in practice and prevent confusion, repetition and gaps in care, it is proposed that nurses will need to learn advanced communication skills that enable them to 'speak the language' of other providers, commissioners and service users.

Policy documents published over the last few years have contained within them common themes for agencies and professionals working together to improve patient care, and increase clinical effectiveness, for example, The New NHS: Modern Dependable (DoH 1997), and the NHS Plan (DoH 2000a). National Service Frameworks (NSFs) in operation take a health and social care perspective on a variety of conditions and recognise that the causes and effects of ill-health require a cross-boundary approach if intervention is to be effective. The National Service Frameworks are designed to raise quality and decrease variations in service delivery by setting standards, defining service models and establishing implementation strategies and performance milestones. More information on National Service Frameworks can be obtained on the website http://www.doh.gov.uk/nsf/about.htm.

The government has articulated a vision of a 'National' Health Service that works closely with other agencies such as housing, education, transport and social services to improve the health of the nation, reduce inequalities and increase the life chances of those who are marginalised or disadvantaged such as those who are disabled, older or suffer from mental health problems. This emphasis on the social factors of ill health has been reinforced by the Government's appointment of a new Minister for Public Health tasked with developing strategies to reduce such health inequalities (Alcock et al 2000).

In order to implement the new National Service Frameworks (Box 11.1) it is imperative that professionals work out with their traditional boundaries and are equipped to be able to communicate with other people and service users in new and participative ways.

Box 11.1 National Service Frameworks for the NHS

Mental Health (1999)
Older People (2001)
Coronary Heart Disease (2000)
Cancer (2000)

National Service Frameworks are intended to set and monitor national standards and service models and put strategies in place that support their implementation. These frameworks are developed with the help of expert reference groups, and it is feasible that some nurses may find themselves in future working on such teams and therefore they need to feel confident to contribute to such an agenda.

Moreover, it is to be appreciated that all parties involved in such complex tasks will not always agree on the goal or the methods to be employed, warranting the use of skilful negotiation. Accordingly, the next section of this chapter will examine in more detail the communication skills that a nurse working, or aspiring to work, in such arenas may wish to consider and extend upon.

KEY COMMUNICATION AREAS FOR ADVANCED AND EFFECTIVE WORKING IN THE NHS

To work effectively in an ever-changing NHS the nurse, in particular those working at a higher level of practice, will need to develop their communication skills to be able to function effectively in four key areas:

◆ collaboration;
◆ partnership;
◆ negotiation;
◆ networking.

These key areas require competent interpersonal communication by nurses who wish to contribute to the 'wider arena' of health care, illustrated in Figure 11.2.

Figure 11.2 presents a systematic view of the areas in which many nurses may find themselves working, and with whom they will have to communicate proficiently. Such an approach will require the nurse to take on a number of roles and styles of communication to achieve a variety of functions each of which are distinct, but have overlapping characteristics and this is shown in Figure 11.3.

These new titles such as networker and partner are increasingly seen in the language and literature of health and social care, however the practical interpretation of them may be less clear. Accordingly, some of these roles and styles are now discussed with examples to illustrate how the nurse may employ and make use of them to improve client care.

COLLABORATION

Collaboration with other agencies, professionals and service users is one of the ways forward clearly envisaged by current health policy, however, to achieve this way of working requires consideration of the skills required, and acknowledgement of the context of the situation in which collaboration is to occur. For individuals working in new roles such as working as nurse consultants, the ability to collaborate is seen as a prerequisite to their success (Stichler 2002).

Heinemann et al (1995) have described collaboration as:

'a complex phenomenon whose definition has remained vague or highly variable. Despite its elusiveness, its essence continues to be sought after as a means of improving working relationships and patient outcomes' (Heinemann et al 1995, p. 2)

Polivka (1995) has proposed that to achieve effective interagency collaboration there needs to be consideration of five major areas, these are shown in Box 11.2 and then discussed.

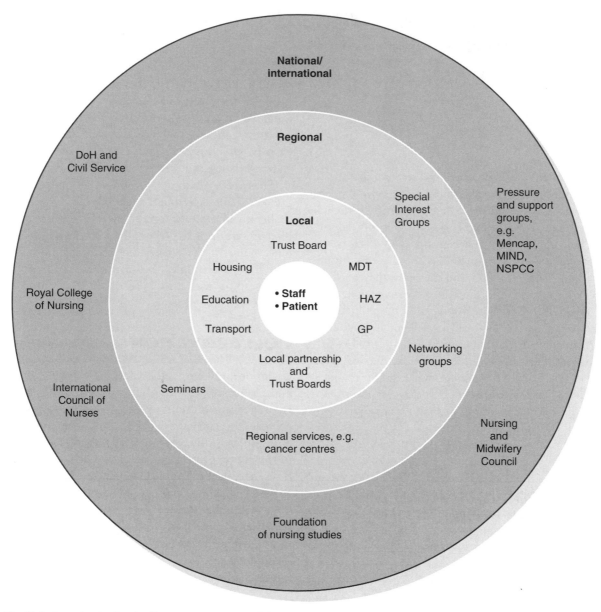

National/international

DoH and Civil Service

Regional

Royal College of Nursing

Special Interest Groups

Pressure and support groups, e.g. Mencap, MIND, NSPCC

Local

Trust Board

Housing   MDT

• **Staff**
• **Patient**

Education   HAZ

Transport   GP

Local partnership and Trust Boards

International Council of Nurses

Seminars

Networking groups

Regional services, e.g. cancer centres

Nursing and Midwifery Council

Foundation of nursing studies

Fig 11.2 Areas involved with effective inter–agency collaboration

Environmental context

The environmental context is described by Polivka (1995) as the major social, political, economic and demographic factors that effect interagency collaboration. Currently, in the United Kingdom, it is reasonable to propose that the 'setting' or environmental context is favourable for collaboration to occur. As previously discussed, nurses and other health care professionals are directed to work in such a manner through policy (DoH 2000, 2001).

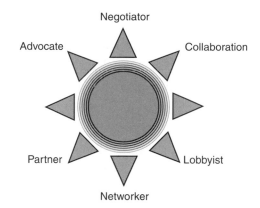

Fig 11.3 Extensions of a nurse's role

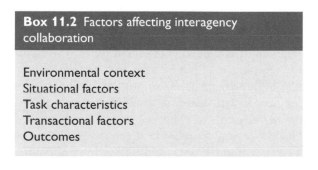

Box 11.2 Factors affecting interagency collaboration

Environmental context
Situational factors
Task characteristics
Transactional factors
Outcomes

This move has been supported by changes within the nursing profession and the UKCC has issued guidance to enable nurses to extend their roles and take on new tasks and assignments (UKCC 1992). It is understood that the new Nursing and Midwifery Council (NMC) will continue to promote such ways of working.

National Service Frameworks (NSFs) such as the one for people with mental health needs (DoH 1999), carry an expectation that staff will work together across interagency boundaries. The NHS Plan (2000), the government's blueprint for the NHS, has highlighted the problem of 'old-fashioned demarcations between staff and barriers between services'.

Situational factors

This is described as the knowledge and awareness that services or organisations have about each other, and that this can be improved if the agencies have shared domains (Polivka 1995). For example the provision of good services for people with learning disabilities requires the collaboration of several groups such as health, social services, transport, housing and education, to communicate and work towards shared goals (DoH 2001). The innovative nurse has been said to be able to work across such boundaries (Hancock 1999) and be able to piece the 'jigsaw' of services together.

Task characteristics

This refers to the extent to which multidisciplinary and multiagency working is required. If the task is complex, that is implementing a National Service Framework, then it is more likely to succeed if more people are able to contribute. However, to be able to do this the nurse must be clear when communicating her role and responsibilities within the team, otherwise a task may become everyone's business but no one person's responsibility. An inherent danger in large teams of mixed professional backgrounds is the ease to make an assumption that a particular task is the job of someone else leading to repetition of the work or, worse, a failure to meet need.

Furthermore, in the initial stages of a collaborative task the process is uncertain and the outcome unpredictable. New projects, or new policy initiatives, usually need people who can articulate with clarity a long-term vision in a way that inspires confidence to other members of the same team who may feel 'frozen' with uncertainty.

Transactional factors

Transactional factors that can influence the effectiveness of collaboration have been described by Polivka (1995) as the policies, committees, shared funds that formalise relationships. Wade (1995) has viewed the sharing of resources to the mutual benefit of all parties as a contributory factor in successful collaboration.

Within the New NHS, provision is made for local partnership boards, pooled budgets, joint committees and implementation teams and will assist members from different agencies to work more closely with one another. For nurses involved in such teams this may mean running committees or writing policies that require communications that are clear and succinct. They may need to know how to set agendas, chair meetings, take minutes, fortunately these skills are easily acquired by way of short in-house training programmes or as part of basic management courses.

Intensity in working relationships and formalised interagency structures are a key feature of the latest government policies such as Valuing People (2001). This is somewhat different to the policies of the past that have tended to make less of an effort to support collaboration that has inevitably led to poor and inconsistent outcomes in levels of care and expenditure (DoH 1999b). Hudson (2000) has described this as a 'paradox' where collaboration between teams and agencies is 'seen as both a problem and solution – failure to work together is the problem, therefore the solution is to work together better!'

A key message here is that any nurse embarking on interagency venture must ensure that enough time and attention is paid to understanding the structure and processes involved (Antrobus & Brown 1997) and making good use of those intended to support communication and the sharing of knowledge. These may include 'time out' days, team briefings, newsletters and group emails in addition to regular meetings and one-to-one discussions.

Outcomes

If outcomes are seen as good and achievable then they become an obvious incentive to collaborate. If positive outcomes can be achieved from interagency and interprofessional working then there are obvious benefits for the patient or service user. Often limited resources make collaboration an imperative (Polivka 1995), and the nurse may

be able to achieve better outcomes by communicating their contribution to patient care with other agencies or groups with similar or overlapping goals in order to maximise effect. Explaining to everyone team achievements is also a way that a nurse can increase team motivation and a sense of purpose. Methods of communicating such messages include distribution of quantitative and qualitative information to all staff such as number of contacts, average length of stay, 'thank you' letters from patients and comments from visits such as those planned by the Commission for Health Improvement (CHI) (see website http://www.chi.gov.uk/).

A case study in collaboration

Jane Smith is a newly appointed nurse consultant for learning disabilities. She has been given the task of improving access to primary health services for people with learning disabilities within a run-down inner city area that is part of a newly formed Health Action Zone. The Primary Health Care Centre within the area is also keen to improve the service and has recently appointed a new GP who is keen to implement policy guidance such as Once a Day (DoH 1999b).

Historically, people with learning disabilities within the area have been poor attendees for both doctor's appointments and well person clinics, despite the fact that they are known to have an increased incidence of physical healthcare needs. Local strategies have been tried in the past but failed and these included extra evening sessions, reminder letters and longer appointment times with the doctor.

 Activity 11.1

If you were Jane how would you use a collaborative approach to solve this problem?

What might be the major issues to consider that prevent people with learning disabilities attending the surgery, and who might be able to help?

How would you explain to others your new role and find out about the roles of other key stakeholders such as the GPs, practice nurse and, most importantly, people with learning disabilities?

Is there an opportunity and incentive for several people/agencies to work together on this issue to achieve common goals.

Collaboration: follow up to Activity 11.1

After spending some time going out and visiting local people and various professionals working in the area, Jane decided that using a collaborative approach to the problem would be the best way forward.

After meeting many people with learning disabilities it became apparent that several problems contributed to them being unable to access primary health care effectively:

1. The area was very run down and crime levels were high and many people with learning disabilities were the targets of harassment and bullying by local youths. This meant that many people were afraid to leave their homes to go to evening surgery and that transport was difficult as bus companies had refused to work after 6 p.m.

2. Many people found the information sent to them about health promotion and special clinics was unhelpful as it was not easy to read and contained a lot of jargon.

3. People who did attend the surgery for clinics such as asthma, felt that they were often pointless as their housing was so damp and difficult to heat that it undermined their efforts. Similarly, those who had attended obesity clinics felt their problems were exacerbated by a lack of opportunity to work or access leisure facilities.

In response Jane initially used the Health Action Zone status as a lever for change. She made contact with local representatives from housing, police, education, employment services and transport. She emphasised the issues raised by service users and highlighted the government and local policies that applied such as Signposts for Success (DoH 1998) and Once a Day (1999b). She held a series of focus groups and 1:1 discussions with key stakeholders in order to formulate and articulate a vision of future services and then developed an action plan for change.

Activities actioned by Jane

◆ Contributing to the future review of the local housing strategy for people with learning disabilities.

◆ Raising the issue of transport with local bus companies resulting in a 'dedicated' bus service being provided to and from the evening surgery.

◆ Discussing the highlighted need for active employment for people with learning disabilities with the directors of supported employment schemes in the area.

◆ Working with service users, speech and language therapist, practice nurses and health promotion departments to provide a range of user friendly materials on topics such as heart disease, exercise and cancer.

◆ Setting up a working party with representatives from local schools, the police, probation and service users to examine ways of reducing bullying and harassment.

◆ Arranging for a social security benefits advisor to be available at targeted clinics such as asthma to ensure people were able to access help with heating etc.

PARTNERSHIP

It has already been stated that the current government is committed to ensuring that staff within the NHS feel they are partners in the running of the organisation (Hancock 1999). This seems a sensible and practical approach to achieving its

Box 11.3

Consensus
Communication
Leadership
Visibility
Involvement
Continuity
Recognition
Strengths

overarching theme of 'inclusiveness' and endeavours to avoid the situation described by Werrett and Carnwell (2001) where poor communication and attitudes are noted to damage relationships between professionals and other agencies and create a situation of 'them and us'.

Hancock in 1999 described her criteria for successful partnerships (Box 11.3). It is proposed that these characteristics afford a framework for nurses who are advancing their practice to work within and when striving to achieve or improve their own partnership working.

Each of these is now briefly discussed.

Consensus

Consensus is described as the values that we share and wish to achieve in relation to patient care (Hancock 1999). The ability to generate a clear vision is vital for nurse leaders (Rippon & Monaghen 2001). Moreover, accepting ownership of the vision requires a nurse to ensure she has listened carefully to the views of all stakeholders and interpreted them accurately. Failure to do so will lead to lack of clarity of purpose, and the danger of misinterpretation.

Communication

Communication of shared values with staff, and effectively articulating the priorities of an organisation is crucial and is as pertinent when undertaken on an individual basis, or as part of group discussions, or whether it is with another staff or with a service user. Wade (1995), in studying the concept of partnership between patient and nurse, has emphasised the common core themes of good communication, interpersonal and negotiation skills.

Nurses in leadership and management positions need to find ways of explaining and sharing the philosophical basis of their work as well as in the operational goals, and in so doing may make use of in-service training days, mentorship and 'walking the floor'.

Individuals also need to explain to other agencies and professionals, such as Social Services, housing, voluntary sector, parents, and most importantly service users of the work of their organisation.

The new NHS will see many nurses imparting information to their partners in care in a variety of ways, including telephone advice lines, and therefore good communication will increasingly become an essential attribute of such staff (Hibberd 1998). This also means that we need to be aware of practical aspects of conversation such as the use of jargon specific to our field or area of work, that may not be understood by other professionals, carers or agencies. Communication by telephone, email and fax is fast and effective but requires a sound knowledge of information technology and the ability to discuss issues without the benefit of nonverbal feedback.

Leadership

Leadership is described as a key characteristic of partnership, as good leaders 'gel' teams together (Hancock 1999). Moreover good leaders have the ability to galvanise individuals to work to a common goal by their 'gift of vision' (Stichler 2002), this is crucial to prevent members of a partnership setting up their own agendas or communicating a conflicting vision in the absence of a clear direction. Large organisations also have to cope with the added problem of messages being 'corrupted' as they are passed through the system. Consequently, leaders need to check and recheck the feedback with staff at 'shop floor' or ward level.

Antrobus and Kitson (1999) have described the skills repertoire required by an individual to consult and work effectively with, and through, others. They described such an individual as needing problem-solving and decision-making skills, as well as knowledge of human processes and communication patterns.

Visibility

Visibility of all the partners including nurses is a prerequisite for a partnership. For nurses increasing their visibility requires them to communicate with the 'public' in its widest sense what they do and what they can contribute to the health and social care agenda (Gordon & Buresh 2001).

Involvement

Involvement is described as consulting users and staff (Hancock 1999). This may take many forms such as traditional meetings, survey, focus groups, one-to-one discussions and team days.

Continuity

Continuity is described as a requirement for 'partners' to have longevity of relationships and appreciation of others skills and knowledge. Unfortunately, changes in staff and local policies as well as the reconfiguration of boundaries can sometimes make the task of creating a stable team difficult. However the use of succession planning, shadowing and mentorship may help in this respect.

Recognition

Recognition of boundaries and enabling everyone to feel valued will encourage greater partnership working. The NHS Plan (DoH 2000a) has positively encouraged the sharing of individual expertise across boundaries. However, to do this we need to communicate our commonalities rather than identify our differences as agencies and professionals. Hibberd (1998) has advocated this approach and a reduction in barriers as being crucial to improve

connections between the primary and secondary care interface.

Strengths

Strengths of each player within a partnership, including nurses, should always be valued. Nursing at all levels is a complex activity and even more so when the nurse is engaged in a consultancy role. Stichler (2002) has described the work of consultancy and highlighted several themes when working with a client (organisation) that are thought relevant to partnership working and these are shown in Box 11.4. Partners, as previously described may be other professionals, i.e. social workers or agencies or charitable service providers (see Box 11.4 for an illustration of the use of partnership).

The consultant needs to be able to understand the partners':

◆ rituals (rewards and recognition protocols, celebrations);
◆ belief systems (mission and value statements);
◆ language (policies and procedures);
◆ structures (organisational structure, approval bodies and approval processes).

NEGOTIATION

If nurses are going to be able to undertake new roles in the wider health and social care arenas such as consultant, nurse practitioner, clinical nurse specialist, then the ability to negotiate is a prerequisite to effective practice. However, being involved in such interactions is quite a new experience as Antrobus and Brown (1997) have stated:

'nursing has historically been identified as relatively naïve in matters outside the immediate province of patient care and has suffered from a lack of real influence in the health policy arena.'

Negotiation may take place in many situations, both informally and formally, however it always

---

Box 11.4 Partnership working (after Stichler 2002)

Illustration of partnership

Jim Jones an experienced Senior Nurse within the care of the elderly directorate of a large general hospital has been asked to work with the manager of a local voluntary organisation to set up a respite care scheme for carers whose partners have debilitating and progressive illness.

On examination of the issues Jim noted that the overarching goal of the two parties involved was the same (keeping families together). The hospital voiced its main aim as improving the health of the patients and their families whilst the voluntary organisation representing carers stated that it wanted to gain breaks for carers and enable some to continue to hold down jobs.

By skilfully communicating the long-term vision of keeping families together, Jim was able to avoid any potential conflict over priorities or responsibilities.

He was able to do this by emphasising the commonalities in 'mission' and valuing the other manager's perspective. When developing the protocols for respite, Jim was mindful to ensure that the language used reflected the belief system of the voluntary organisation and the service user. Where possible clinical terms and jargon were avoided and a 'common language' was agreed, this involved agreeing to write all guidance and policies in plain English. Meetings to discuss progress were held in mutually agreed venues that encouraged user involvement such as the local library and were co-chaired.

Lastly, Jim made sure that when taking the protocols and bid for finance forward he was well briefed on the approval process and planning cycle of the voluntary organisation as well as the NHS.

---

involves good communication skills. Being able to negotiate a contract at a meeting between agencies, and even negotiate on behalf of nursing on a piece of legislation or policy requires the same preparation and clarity about what is needed and the purpose of the meeting. Fletcher (1998) has offered a list of questions to assist the 'would be' health service negotiator make sense of the negotiation process and this is shown in Box 11.5.

Although not traditionally taught, negotiation skills are vital to nurses working in new and 'uncharted territory' (Wade 1995). The ability to negotiate is essential to ensure that they achieve their stated goals and intended outcomes. Many new roles such as the 'modern matron' and 'nurse consultant' require the nurse to influence policy, not just locally but also at national level. Antrobus and Brown (1997) have stated:

'policy can best be understood as the product of a bargaining process between a limited number of groups each one interdependent upon the other, within a wider social and

economic context' (Antrobus & Brown 1997, p. 5).

So, how do nurses bargain? How do they negotiate with others to gain the most benefit for their client group or service?

Fletcher (1998) has described negotiation as 'people talking'. He stated that to undertake successful negotiation we need to be aware of the written, verbal and nonverbal signals one is sending. For example a poorly constructed report may repel the receiver, whereas a well-written and clear commentary may invite negotiation.

Using the words and language of the recipient (see Chapter 1) may reinforce a sense of sameness between 'you and them' and foster allegiance. You will need to be able to communicate clearly and listen carefully and judge the 'mood' of an encounter to enable you to alter your tone according to response, signs of boredom or agitation or even anger. It is worth remembering that the nurse acting as a consultant may have to present findings that are controversial to an audience, and therefore

Box 11.5 Making sense of the negotiation process (adapted from Fletcher 1998)

Who am I and what am I doing here?	This asks you to think about the role that you are undertaking in this particular meeting and your own underlying values and attitudes. For instance you may be representing the NHS Trust for whom you work as a representative of a team or you may be representing yourself as an individual practitioner.
What do I want?	Be clear about your objectives and your 'bottom line'. Know what is the most desirable and least desirable outcome. When representing others ensure you have canvassed views thoroughly.
What am I prepared to give to get what I want?	This may be nothing, or may be the commitment of time or services or the relinquishment of a traditional role.
Who are they and what are they doing here?	Consider their role, agenda, motives for negotiating, how much power they have and what they stand to gain from the meeting? Who is watching them? What are their cultural and organisational influences?
What do they want?	Try and work out their objectives and their 'bottom line'.
What are they prepared to give to get what they want?	This is important because the thing they wish to give may be your main goal and they may not be aware of it! You may need to think laterally as they may be prepared to help with an unrelated but equally difficult problem.
How do I prepare the ground?	Analyse the strengths and weakness of all parties involved in the negotiation including you. Remember it is not a competition; you are looking for common ground that might help you both achieve the objective.
How do I manage the exchange?	Consider the timing of the meeting, do not allow yourself to be rushed – ask for an adjournment if things take an unexpected turn. Don't waffle and ensure you actively listen to the other parties' responses. Remember not to use jargon or specialist language that may exclude others. Be aware of body language and nonverbal messages.
How do I assess the result?	Go back to your objectives; did you get what you wanted? Did you find the common ground? Was mutual agreement reached?

require advanced presentation skills to ensure a meeting remains constructive (Stichler 2002).

Nurses may have to use negotiation skills in a variety of settings and to achieve a variety of outcomes. As a member of a Local Implementation Board or Primary Care Trust a nurse may be negotiating topics for inclusion into Health Improvement Programmes (HIMPs), Joint Investment Plans (JIPs) and Health Action Zones (HAZs). There will often be many competing and conflicting priorities proposed by various professionals and agencies, and the skill of the nurse will ensure she is able to negotiate the best position possible for the client group.

Some nurses working in new, and often ground-breaking, areas will sometimes need to negotiate pay and conditions, workloads and even balance the needs of more than one organisation; for example lecturer practitioners are responsible to both a university and their NHS employer. Negotiation, selling and conflict management skills are crucial when the views of the nurse are fundamentally different to those of the organisation management or leadership in force (Stichler 2002).

Current nursing leadership urges nurses to be involved in influencing health policy and strategy and ensure that plans for the health service are based on the best advice available (Mullally 2001).

Influencing the political agenda may take many forms. One method of meeting, negotiating and influencing policy makers is 'grassroots lobbying' described by Ober (1999). This involves nurses or other health care professions using their communication and political skills to obtain changes in legislation. For example a nurse's special interest group may have noticed a funding problem in relation to a local service or that nurses' views have not being canvassed in relation to a policy that is still in the draft stage. If you are invited to a meeting with a civil servant or Member of Parliament or even attending a Board meeting it is worth studying the advice offered by Ober (1999), shown in Box 11.6.

NETWORKING

Networking is primarily concerned with interacting with others in an effective and assisting manner. The nurse should not see networking as something that nurses at 'higher' levels of practice undertake but as something that all nurses should engage in. The clouding of boundaries between professionals and agencies calls for more use of networking as we share increasingly common problems and responsibilities for the same issues. Networking may help us to learn from the mistakes or successes of others in similar roles or it may gain us support and mentorship to enable us to find our own solution to a unique problem.

Networking should be seen as a reciprocal relationship with each party standing to gain from the interaction over time. Networking may take a variety of forms each involving skilful communication, these have been articulated by the UKCC and are shown in Box 11.7.

Box 11.6 Advice for meetings

Never bring a large group of people to a meeting without asking beforehand;
Always be punctual;
Instead of the whole document – try to leave an executive summary;
Avoid health jargon;
Do not flood the legislators office with faxes, emails, letters;
Never give false or misleading information.

Adapted from Ober (1999).

Box 11.7 Variations of networking

Formal – planned activity within a team or department.
Informal – as an unplanned contact at a seminar, conference, meeting or training course.
Organised – by others such as a local or regional symposium or national or international conference.
Localised and self generated.
Thematic – specifically arranged to discuss a particular issue or clinical problem such as vaccination programmes.
Reactive and possibly short lived – to look at a new government policy or guidance and discuss its implications.

Adapted from UKCC (2000).

In order to network effectively the nurse will need to be able to communicate with other people in a variety of ways, and this will include the following.

Face-to-face

In the main, most networking will be a process of one individual meeting another and sharing information. However, actively engaging another person in the process may require you to undertake some preparation and planning. You will firstly need to ask yourself 'Is this the right person to approach to resolve a particular issue?'. Demonstrating a lack of knowledge about the other person's role and involvement in a project is unlikely to motivate them to engage with you at the outset! It is vital to be clear about the purpose of the meeting especially if the encounter is likely to be brief. Do you primarily want to share your work, or do you want to find out how they achieved success?

At the first meeting give a brief résumé of your role and articulate your issue/s to the other person in an informal but clear manner, in order to enable them to highlight the parts of their work that they feel will be of most help or interest. Emphasise areas of commonality between roles and responsibilities and balance problems with achievements – you do not want to appear to be constantly moaning or alternatively, bragging!

Newsletters and bulletins

Most organisations today have some form of newsletter that can be widely distributed and can be a valuable source of networking with others. There are various ways to take advantage of this media:

◆ Asking for assistance with a problem or issue – for example you may be trying to raise funds and asking for volunteers with similar interests to join in.

◆ Celebrating an achievement – you may wish to tell others of your team's success in reaching a target or goal. This not only serves to motivate the team but also to let other teams know it can be done, and how to do it.

◆ Highlighting an emergent issue or concern – it may be that your team has observed an increase in a particular phenomenon, for example accidents in children under 5, and you might want to know if other teams have also noticed similar problems within their locality.

◆ Sharing news – you may wish to inform others who have the same or a similar job of a piece of news that affects everyone. For example a community nurse in one locality may wish to tell all community nurses across a Trust about a change in guidance or policy.

◆ Advertising events – informing others of forthcoming networking opportunities such as local seminars, workshops and conferences.

Use of information technology

Increasingly, nurses are using IT to help them keep in touch with others and share ideas. IT can be used in a variety of ways and has many advantages over traditional forms of communication such as newsletters, in that it is quicker, the news is more up to date and the process can be interactive with others.

Many nursing organisations and special interest groups have their own website to enable nurses to communicate with each other. 'Chat rooms' enable a dialogue to be facilitated and ideas debated and commented upon. Many websites have 'useful links' to other sites of similar interest and this will allow the nurse to build up a more extensive network.

Importantly, governmental departments have website and email addresses which nurses can access. New policies and guidance are frequently published on such sites and often in draft form to enable practitioners to comment and offer their experiences. Nurses must make use of such opportunities to shape both the profession and patient care as well as positively embracing the opportunity to engage interactively with policymakers.

Many special interest groups now have their own website and email addresses where people from similar fields like mental health nursing, can network and communicate their ideas and can be found through professional organisations such as the Royal College of Nursing website – http://www. rcn.org.uk.

When using emails and chatrooms it is worth remembering some of the basic rules of communication, that is, be clear, be polite and avoid the use of jargon. You will obviously not be able to pick up on nonverbal signals and so will need to carefully concentrate on the words used by the sender in order to pick up the tone of the conversation. This can be done in much the same way as one would assess the tone of a letter for example ask yourself:

◆ Is this conversation flowing or abrupt?
◆ Are people using the same language or are they at crossed purposes?
◆ Are the other person's answers characteristically yes or no all the time?
◆ Is the other person offering anything, or is it all one way?

Of course it pays to remember that IT interactions are, by nature, brief and not a place to elaborate a thesis, however, they should encourage interaction and reciprocation.

Video and teleconferencing

The thought of being on camera often terrifies most people, and in particular many nurses! However, in a world where increasingly, debate takes place on national and international platforms, they are invaluable forms of communication. Many health care organisations are geographically spread over wide areas, with many bases and it makes sense to be able to network from one's own base from time to time, rather than always meet at one venue. Benefits of using this media for networking include:

◆ saving on time and cost of transport;
◆ ability to interact with people locally, regionally, nationally and internationally;
◆ video conferencing allows participants to pick up on nonverbal as well as verbal messages, which can be particularly helpful, when the topic of discussion is complex or contentious;
◆ video and teleconferencing often brings 'richness' to a debate that would not be possible to

facilitate by any other method. For example how would you be able to draw in the comments of a nurse working in France in a contemporaneous manner unless you brought her to the meeting?

Networking groups

You may decide that it is worthwhile establishing a networking group and meeting on a regular basis to discuss issues and share ideas. Before you set up your group it may be wise to make checks in a number of areas, these might include:

◆ Checking if there is an existing similar group in the area and consider joining that one – setting up another group may dilute membership across groups as well as causing confusion, antagonism and competition.
◆ Asking around to see who might be interested in joining and elicit their help and support.
◆ Check that your 'line manager' would be supportive of staff attending meetings and forums.

CONCLUSION

Developing the skills to communicate with the 'wider world' is a continuous and dynamic process. The further one's career progresses the greater the opportunity to network and consult grows. Emphasis has been placed on the need for the modern practitioner to work in partnership and collaboration and to seek to articulate a clear vision and identify common ground that may facilitate rather than impede success.

This chapter has further highlighted a number of roles and methods of communication to enable and empower nurses to participate as members of the health care arena.

To respond effectively and deliver care responsively nurses need to develop a range of interpersonal techniques and make best use of the range of technology available. Most importantly they should remember their basic training and the need to consult service users before all else.

REFERENCES

Alcock C, Payne S, Sullivan M 2000 Introducing social policy. Prentice Hall, Harlow

Antrobus S, Brown S 1997 The impact of the Commissioning Agenda upon nursing: a proactive approach to influencing health policy. Journal of Advanced Nursing 25(2): 309–315

Antrobus S, Kitson A 1999 Nursing leadership: influencing and shaping health policy and nursing practice. Journal of Advanced Nursing 29(3): 746–753

Department of Health 1997 The new NHS. Modern, dependable. Cm 3807. The Stationary Office, London

Department of Health 1998 Signposts for success in commissioning and providing health services for people with learning disabilities. Department of Health NHSE, Wetherby

Department of Health 1999a National service framework for mental health: modern standards and service models. The Stationary Office, London

Department of Health 1999b Once a day. Department of Health, Wetherby

Department of Health 2000a The NHS plan: a plan for investment. A plan for reform. Cm 4818-1. HMSO, London

Department of Health 2000b National service framework for coronary heart disease: modern standards and service models. The Stationary Office, London

Department of Health 2000c The NHS cancer plan: a plan for investment, a plan for reform. The Stationary Office, London

Department of Health 2001 Valuing people: a new strategy for learning disability for the 21st century. HMSO, London

Fletcher K 1998 Negotiation for health and social services professionals. Jessica Kingsley Publications, London

Gordon S, Buresh B 2001 Speak out loud for nursing. Nursing Management 7(10): 14–17

Hancock C 1999 Partnership; The challenge for nursing (lecture). Nursing Management 6(3): 33–37

Heinneman E, Lee JL, Cohen J 1995 Collaboration: a concept analysis. Journal of Advanced Nursing 21(1): 103–109

Hibberd PA 1998 The primary/secondary interface. Cross-boundary teamwork – the missing link for seamless care? Journal of Clinical Nursing 7(3): 274–282

Hudson B 2000 Inter-agency collaboration – a sceptical view. In: Brechin A, Brown H, Eby MA Critical practice in health & social care. Sage, London

Mullally S 2001 Leadership and politics (LPNS lecture). Nursing Management 8(4): 21–27

Ober S 1999 Making grassroots action effective. AORN Journal 70(4): 699–701

Polivka BJ 1995 A conceptual model for community interagency collaboration. Image – the Journal of Nursing Scholarship 27(2): 110–115

Rippon S, Monaghen A 2001 Clinical leadership embracing a bold new agenda. Nursing Management 8(6): 6–9

Stichler JF 2002 The nurse as consultant. Nursing Administration Quarterly 26(2): 52–68

UKCC 1992 The scope of professional practice. UKCC, London

UKCC 2000 Networking in learning disability nursing. A guide. UKCC, London

Wade S 1995 Partnership in care: a critical review. Nursing Standard 9(48): 29–32

Werrett J, Carnwell R 2001 The primary and secondary care interface: the educational needs of nursing staff for the provision of seamless care. Journal of Advanced Nursing 34(5): 629–638

Index